GROWING PAINS

GROWING PAINS

CHILDHOOD ILLNESS IN IRELAND, 1750–1950

EDITORS
ANNE MAC LELLAN
ALICE MAUGER

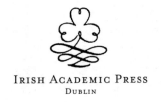

IRISH ACADEMIC PRESS
DUBLIN

First published in 2013 by Irish Academic Press

8 Chapel Lane,
Sallins,
Co. Kildare,
Ireland

www.iap.ie

British Library Cataloguing in Publication Data
An entry can be found on request

ISBN 978 0 7165 3160 9 (cloth)
ISBN 978 0 7165 3173 9 (paper)
ISBN 978 0 7165 3205 7 (Ebook)

Library of Congress Cataloging-in-Publication Data
An entry can be found on request

Printed in Ireland by SPRINT-print

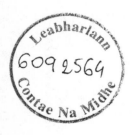

This book is dedicated to Professor Conor Ward, distinguished paediatrician and medical historian, who has been a staunch supporter of this project from its first incarnation as a workshop through to the completed volume. His encouragement and generosity with his time and expertise is greatly appreciated.

CONTENTS

FOREWORD

Lindsey Earner-Byrne

Growing Pains, a study of childhood illness in Ireland between 1750 and 1950, represents the initiative and dedication of two scholars from the Centre for the History of Medicine in Ireland at the School of History and Archives, University College Dublin: Anne Mac Lellan and Alice Mauger, who have ensured that the energy of a workshop has left a lasting imprint. As editors they have brought together an impressive selection of contributors from UCD, the University of Ulster, St Patrick's College, Dublin City University, NUI Maynooth, and Trinity College Dublin, whose essays collectively offer the reader one of the first detailed considerations of the history of childhood illness in Ireland. This volume covers a period when one-third of Ireland's children were killed by smallpox (1700s) and twenty per cent of infants died before the first birthday (1800s): if you survived childhood, the prospect of losing your own children was not just a fear, but an ever-present reality until the 1950s.

The contributors have used a wide variety of sources including institutional records, government publications, correspondence, contemporary medical books and oral history. This has resulted in a rich collection that offers fresh historical perspectives, for example, the essay on Irish child survivors of the Spanish Flu (1918-1919) uses oral history to explore the social impact of the disease. The survivors paint vivid pictures of 'black Belgian horses pulling hearses for days' in Belfast and challenge us to find new ways of accessing the patient experience.

At the beginning of the twentieth century tuberculosis was the third leading cause of death in children, and two essays address the politics behind the cure, the role of pioneers such as Dorothy Price and unsung heroes like Sister Mary Finbar of Cappagh Hospital. Sister Mary Finbar was recalled by the childhood sufferers of bone and joint TB during the 1940s for her kindness and love during their long and emotionally sterile periods of institutional confinement which reminds us of the emotional impact of illness on its victims.

While these essays point to the major impact an individual could have on the experience and treatment of patients, like Dr Ella Webb and her work for children with rickets, there is also the recurring theme of the emergence of institutions. For example, the development of children's hospital services in the early nineteenth century, in particular the Dublin Institution for the Diseases of Children (est. 1822) and the debates that ensued regarding in-patient hospital accommodation for children. The dreaded workhouse also features in an exploration of its treatment of the 95,000 children who contracted childhood ophthalmia while inmates during the Great Famine and the many others who suffered from the 'falling sickness' or epilepsy that were left to die within its walls. The study of the treatment of children with syphilis examines the mingling of prejudice and compassion. The reader is also challenged to reconsider the historical construction of reformatory and industrial schools and include in our final analysis the original intentions behind these institutions to reform rather than punish body and mind.

The overarching narrative of how changing concepts of childhood illness and childhood itself informed attitudes, care, policy and politics, is explored in every essay through a detailed analysis of a specific topic. While each of these essays tells their own intricate tale, certain themes reappear: the role of the carer, the potential power of determined individuals, the emergence of institutions and the impact of poverty. There is little doubt that the editors' hope will be realised and this volume will act as an inspiration for future research into the history of childhood illnesses in Ireland.

Lindsey Earner-Byrne
Lecturer in Modern Irish History, School of History and Archives, UCD.

List of Figures and Tables

Figure 1: Children Inoculated in the Dublin Workhouse and Foundling Hospital, 1789–96.

Figure 2: Number of Admissions and Outcome of Children's Smallpox and Inoculation in the Dublin Workhouse and Foundling Hospital, 1789–96.

Figure 3: Agents Appointed by the Sutton Family to 'Regulate and Extend their Art over the Kingdom of Ireland'.

Figure 4: Selected Dublin Publications Relative to Children's Healthcare in Eighteenth-Century Ireland.

Figure 5: Towns where the Ophthalmia Epidemic was Most Severe.

Table 1: Number and Percentages of Admissions and Deaths of Patients in the Westmoreland Lock Hospital, 1 January to 31 December 1817 and 1 January to 31 December 1819.

Table 2: Syphilitic Infants Born in the Westmoreland Lock Hospital, 1877–83.

Table 3: Figures for Admissions, Deaths and Births at the Westmoreland Lock Hospital, 1885–1900.

Table 4: Undiseased and Diseased Mothers and Infants Admitted to the Westmoreland Lock Hospital, 1886–92.

Table 5: Incidence of Ophthalmia in Irish Workhouses, 1849–53.

Table 6: Figures for Patients Admitted to the Children's Sunshine Home, 1928–46.

Table 7: Annual X-Rays taken at Graymount and Greenisland.

Table 8: Complications of Spinal Tuberculosis Before and After the Use of Chemotherapy.

List of Plates

1. 'Vertical Mesial Section of Body of Boy aged Six Years' and 'Vertical Mesial Section of Body of Girl aged Thirteen', in J. Symington, *The Topographical Anatomy of the Child* (London: Bailliere, Tindall & Cox, 1887), Plates I and II, pp.9, 11.
Reproduced by kind permission of the Royal College of Physicians of Ireland.

2. Line Drawing of the Moy Mell Children's Guild, Temple Street, in *Twenty-Eighth Annual Report of the Children's Hospital Temple Street and Report of the Moy Mell Children's Guild* (Dublin, 1901).
Courtesy of Temple Street Children's University Hospital.

3. Photograph of R.T. Evanson and H. Maunsell, *A Practical Treatise on the Management and Diseases of Children*, 3rd edn (Dublin: Fannin, 1840).
Reproduced by kind permission of the Royal College of Physicians of Ireland.

4. Undated photograph of the Children's Sunshine Home, Stillorgan (Overend Archive, Airfield Trust, Dublin).
Reproduced by kind permission of Kathy Purcell, Director, Airfield Trust.

5. J. Connolly, Watercolour Illustration of the Case of J. Courtney, aged 11. Illustration shows Courtney's back, which is covered in a rash caused by syphilis in the mid-nineteenth century (Royal College of Physicians of Ireland, MI/1/9).
Reproduced by kind permission of the Royal College of Physicians of Ireland.

6. Kevin – 13 months at St Ultan's Hospital, 23 April 1923 (Royal College of Physicians of Ireland, St Ultan's Hospital photographic album 1919-29, (SU/8/3/1).
Reproduced by kind permission of the Royal College of Physicians of Ireland.

7. Doctors and Patients at St Ultan's Hospital, 30 May 1924 (Royal College of Physicians of Ireland, St Ultan's Hospital photograph album 1919–29, SU/8/3/1).
Reproduced by kind permission of the Royal College of Physicians of Ireland.

8. 'Senior Girls – Surgical Cases': Patients at Stannington Sanatorium, Morpeth, Northumberland, the first British sanatorium for tuberculosis illustrating immobilisation techniques for tuberculous children.
Reproduced by kind permission of the Wellcome Library, London.

9. 'The Diagnosis of Smallpox': illustrates the appearance of smallpox in a small child (T.F. Ricketts, Casell & Company, 1908).
Reproduced by kind permission of the Wellcome Library, London.

10. 'Male and Female Children with Rickets – Side View, c. 1901', in Masson and Cie (eds), *Nouvelle Iconographie de la Salpétrière; Clinique des Maladies du Système Nerveus* (Paris: Libraires de l'Academie de Medecine, c. 1901), Tome XIV, Plate XLIV.
Reproduced by kind permission of the Wellcome Library, London.

11. Clemens von Pirquet and a patient.
Reproduced by kind permission of the Wellcome Library, London.

Acknowledgements

This volume is largely the child of a workshop held in University College Dublin (UCD), in December 2010, entitled 'Paediatric Diseases throughout the Ages: New Perspectives'. This workshop was convened by Wellcome Trust-funded doctoral students Anne Mac Lellan and Alice Mauger. It was hosted by the Centre for the History of Medicine in Ireland (CHOMI) and funded by the Wellcome Trust. We would like to thank the Wellcome Trust for supporting the doctoral studies of the editors in addition to kindly funding the workshop. We would like to thank CHOMI for hosting the workshop and we are grateful to all of the participants who made the workshop such a lively and useful forum. Presenters were postgraduates or early-career historians with the exception of the keynote speaker Professor Conor Ward. The success of this lively workshop was such that one of the speakers, Jean M. Walker, suggested an edited collection might be germane. A theme and contributors were agreed.

We would like to thank all of the authors who have revised and responded to comments with grace and patience. We are indebted to a generous group of readers who read and commented on one and sometimes more chapters. These include Professor Greta Jones, Professor James Kelly, Professor Eoin O'Brien FRCP, Professor Conor Ward, Dr Sarah-Anne Buckley, Dr Clara Cullen, Dr Brendan Kelly, Dr Dympna McLoughlin, Dr Ian Miller and Dr Mary Muldowney. We are extremely grateful to Dr Ian Miller for his unwavering attention, support and guidance at every stage of this lengthy project. We say a heartfelt thank you to Dr Catherine Cox, Director of the UCD Centre for the History of Medicine in Ireland, who supported the workshop. She also attentively supervised the doctoral studies of both editors and for this we are very grateful. Lisa Hyde of Irish Academic Press has been unflappable throughout the process of guiding this book to fruition. For this, we say a heartfelt thank you. We are also very grateful to Dr Lindsey Earner-Byrne for her enthusiasm about the book and for writing the foreword.

The encouragement of Dr Clara Cullen and Dr Margaret Ó hÓgartaigh is also greatly appreciated. A veritable army of archivists and librarians have provided information to the contributors. Their co-operation and assistance has been invaluable.

The wonderful illustrations in this volume were sourced in the library and archives of the Royal College of Physicians of Ireland (RCPI), the archives of the Children's University Hospital (CUH), Temple Street, Dublin and the Wellcome Trust Images Collection, London. The cover photograph is from the CUH. We would like to thank Harriet Wheelock, archivist at the RCPI, who located many of the images and supported the project. Barry Kennerk of the CUH was equally enthusiastic and generous in his provision of images while the Wellcome Images service was prompt and professional.

Notes on Contributors

Gabrielle Ashford graduated from St Patrick's College, Dublin City University in November 2012. Her PhD, 'Childhood: Studies in the History of Children in Eighteenth-Century Ireland', incorporating the digital humanities project 'Irish Children in Eighteenth-Century Schools and Institutions', was funded by An Foras Feasa. Gabrielle tutors in St Patrick's College and is a part-time lecturer in digital humanities on the History masters programme. Her research interests embrace eighteenth-century childhood, Irish emigration, and local and family research.

June Cooper graduated from NUI Maynooth in September 2009 with a PhD entitled 'The Protestant Orphan Society, 1828–1928'. June is an independent scholar whose main research interests are child welfare, paediatric medical care, the family, women's history, and religious minorities in nineteenth- and twentieth-century Ireland.

Philomena Gorey is in the final year of her PhD entitled 'From Ecclesiastical Regulation to State Registration: The Regulation of Irish Midwives c. 1650–1918' at University College Dublin. Her research interests include the changing regulatory parameters within which the midwife worked over the period and the development of man-midwifery in eighteenth-century Dublin. Her chapter, entitled 'Managing Midwifery in Dublin: Practice and Practitioners, 1700–1800', is included in Margaret Preston and Margaret Ó hÓgartaigh (eds), *Gender and Medicine in Ireland* (New York: Syracuse University Press, 2012).

Laura Kelly undertook her IRCHSS-funded PhD entitled 'Irish Medical Women c. 1880s–1920s: The Origins, Education and Careers of Early Women Medical Graduates from Irish Institutions' at the Department of

History, NUI Galway (2007–10). The monograph of her thesis was published by Manchester University Press in 2012. Laura is currently an Irish Research Council Postdoctoral Research Fellow at the Centre for the History of Medicine at University College Dublin (2012–14). Her current project is entitled "'Merry Boys and Winsome Women': Education, Experiences and the Shaping of the Professional Identity of Irish Medical Students, c. 1800–1950'. Laura's research interests include the history of medical education, the medical profession, and women in medicine in nineteenth- and twentieth-century Ireland.

Susan Kelly was awarded a PhD from the University of Ulster in December 2008 for her dissertation entitled "'Suffer the Little Children': Childhood Tuberculosis in the North of Ireland, c. 1865 to 1965'. Susan is an associate member of the Centre for the History of Medicine in Ireland at the University of Ulster. The main focus of her research has been on childhood illness in Ireland in the nineteenth and twentieth centuries. She has a particular interest in oral history.

Anne Mac Lellan graduated from the School of History and Archives, University College Dublin, in December 2011 with a Wellcome Trust-funded PhD thesis entitled 'That Curable and Preventable Disease: Dr Dorothy Price and the Eradication of Tuberculosis in Ireland, 1930–1960'. Anne is the director of research at the Rotunda Hospital, Dublin. She also lectures on a part-time basis in the National College of Art and Design. She is the winner of the RCPI History of Medicine Research Award 2012.

Alice Mauger is a Wellcome Trust-funded doctoral student at the Centre for the History of Medicine in Ireland (University College Dublin). Her doctoral thesis is entitled "'The Great Class Which Lies Between': Provision for the Non-Pauper Insane in Nineteenth-Century Ireland'. Alice's first article, "'Confinement of the Higher Orders': The Social Role of Private Lunatic

Asylums in Ireland, c. 1820–60', was published in *Journal of the History of Medicine and Allied Sciences* in April 2012. Her research interests include history of psychiatry, and medicine in nineteenth- and twentieth-century Ireland.

Ian Miller is an Irish Research Council Government of Ireland Postdoctoral Fellow based at the Centre for the History of Medicine in Ireland (University College Dublin). His monograph *A Modern History of the Stomach: Gastric Illness, Medicine and British Society, 1800–1950* was published by Pickering & Chatto in 2011. He is currently finalising a second monograph, provisionally entitled *Reforming Food in Post-Famine Ireland: Medicine, Science and Improvement, 1845-1922*, to be published with Manchester University Press. Ian has also published widely on the history of medicine and diet in nineteenth- and twentieth-century Britain and Ireland.

Ida Milne was awarded a PhD from Trinity College Dublin in July 2011 for her dissertation 'The 1918–19 Influenza Pandemic in Ireland: A Leinster Perspective'. She is a founder member and director of the Oral History Network of Ireland and uses oral history to explore her main research interest: the history of pandemic influenza, and her other research interests, including welfare and public health, the working lives of medical professionals and newspaper history.

Jean M. Walker was awarded a PhD in 2010 from the Department of Modern History at NUI Maynooth with a thesis on the Westmoreland Lock Hospital, Dublin, and the Treatment of Syphilis, 1792–1900. She currently teaches electives at NUI Maynooth on gender and identity in Irish history. Jean's research interests include social history of health and gendered history.

Conor Ward is Professor Emeritus of Paediatrics in University College Dublin. He is a distinguished paediatric cardiologist and is eponymous with the Ward-Romano syndrome, the disorder of cardiac rhythm that he first described. In retirement, he enrolled as a mature student of medical history and was awarded a PhD in 2000. His biography of John Langdon Down was published by the Royal Society of Medicine Press and received an award from the British Society of Authors. He is a founder member of the British Association for the History of Paediatrics and Child Health and has written extensively on medical history. The main focus of his research has been on the hospital care of children in the Victorian era.

Introduction: Contexts of Childhood Illness in Ireland[1]

Alice Mauger and Anne Mac Lellan

'*Your* child is terminally ill. ...' Few phrases evoke such complex emotional responses. For parents, childhood illness of any kind is feared and highly distressing. Outside the realm of immediate family, friends, neighbours and even healthcare professionals can struggle to come to terms with the serious illness of a child. The death of a child leaves in its wake feelings of helplessness and despair, while caring for a chronically ill child prompts a great deal of soul-searching.[2] In recent centuries these responses have been grounded in a universal acceptance of the sanctity of childhood.

Historically, concerns over child health and welfare have been closely informed by shifting conceptions of childhood. As Hugh Cunningham has argued, in the eighteenth century, childhood was transformed as it became viewed 'not as a preparation for something else, whether adulthood or heaven, but as a stage of life to be valued in its own right'.[3] In the Irish context, Gabrielle Ashford has identified a similar growth in the recognition of children as individuals requiring attention and care distinct from adults.[4] Internationally, the nineteenth century witnessed debates on issues such as child labour and parental cruelty.[5] These were often articulated in terms of saving the child for the enjoyment of childhood and drew heavily on ideals of Romanticism.[6] Heightened sensitivity towards child welfare resulted in a dramatic increase in philanthropic and state intervention in this arena, while the institutionalization of certain social groups of children gathered momentum.[7] In Ireland the Great Famine resulted in a surge in the number of children accommodated in workhouses; in 1850 there were almost 120,000, a figure that reduced to just over 18,000 by the mid-1860s.[8] In addition, various religious organizations, both Catholic and Protestant, attended to the needs of increasing numbers of orphans.[9] The late nineteenth century saw the establishment of the Dublin Aid Society, a philanthropic organization concerned with protecting children from physical and sexual abuse. In 1900 this became known as the National Society for the Prevention of Cruelty to Children, Dublin and District Branch (NSPCC).[10]

In early twentieth-century Britain, according to Hilary Marland and Marijke Gijswijt-Hofstra, 'the condition and status of the child was closely bound up with concerns of national efficiency and citizenship', reflecting broader apprehensions about the fitness of the nation in a period leading up to war.[11] Anna Davin has aligned these anxieties with British imperialism and a new imagining of 'the value of a healthy and numerous population as a national resource'.[12] Marland and Gijswijt-Hofstra have suggested that the topic of child health in the twentieth century has 'far stronger links with notions of "fitness" and "welfare" than with illness *per se*'.[13] They link this to a decline in epidemic diseases and infant mortality rates from around 1900 and identify a consequent shift in focus towards longer-term health issues.[14] Ireland provides more complex scope for the exploration of child health issues. Similar to Britain, growing concerns about national deterioration brought to the fore discussion of how best to promote the physical and psychological stamina of the rising generation.[15] However, in the Irish context, these debates tended not to be linked to imperial or colonial objectives. In fact, critics of British state policies for Ireland (characterized by an absence of legislation for school meals and medical inspection until later than England) accused the state of deliberately subjugating, rather than strengthening, the bodies of the nation, as argued by Ian Miller.[16] Nationalists, in turn, implied that these policies were responsible for the poor health of Irish children and the perpetuation of national physical and psychological decline.[17]

In addition to the clear emergence of concerns surrounding national fitness and children in the Irish context, child healthcare professionals were also faced with the persistence of higher infant mortality rates and higher mortality from childhood diseases than other countries, including Britain.[18] In terms of child welfare, Maria Luddy suggests that 'disquiet over high levels of infant mortality, the nourishment of the poor and street-trading children, among other concerns' also stimulated greater interest during this era.[19] Concerns about diseases such as tuberculosis and rickets persisted well into the twentieth century, prompting both philanthropic and medical action.[20] The issue of child health in twentieth-century Ireland may thus be cast in multiple frameworks. On the one hand, Irish fears about national deterioration echoed those expressed in Britain, albeit couched in very different political rhetoric. On the other, poor living conditions, deficient diets and overcrowding in Ireland's urban centres – often worse than in other major cities in the British Isles – meant a continuing need to tackle debilitating and even life-threatening illnesses in children. This resulted in a duality in health, welfare and medical approaches in Ireland that was seemingly less marked in other countries.

Although historical research on child welfare issues such as these has burgeoned in recent decades, Alysa Levene has noted that studies of the medical care of children have developed 'only in fits and starts'.[21] Seminal collections such as Roger Cooter's *In the Name of the Child* and Marland and Gijswijt-Hofstra's *Cultures of Child Health* have emphasized health and welfare rather than medical practice across the late nineteenth and twentieth centuries. Despite a growth in historiographical attention directed at child health, much remains to be done. Levene has recently argued that exploring how practitioners and parents treated sick children could reveal much about attitudes towards children in general.[22] Marland and Gijswijt-Hofstra have suggested that the history of the sick child warrants more attention.[23] Furthermore, very few studies have emerged on specific diseases of childhood, how they were treated and how they were perceived.

In Ireland the historical study of childhood illness remains relatively uncharted territory.[24] In 2010 Catherine Cox and Maria Luddy noted the 'current vibrancy' in Irish medical history while highlighting a lack of knowledge about 'Irish attitudes to sick children, their care within homes or within institutions'.[25] Although internationally the history of childhood is a vast field, boasting such highly regarded studies as Cunningham's *Children and Childhood in Western Society*, offerings relating to Ireland have been comparatively meagre.[26] In 2009 a special issue of *Éire-Ireland* was dedicated to children, childhood and Irish society. In its introduction, Maria Luddy and James Smith highlighted that 'we still know very little about how Irish society understood childhood or children, or how those concepts evolved and changed over the centuries'.[27] A dedicated analysis of childhood illness in Ireland thus bridges gaps in our knowledge of the social, cultural and medical history of childhood in Ireland. This volume brings together a collection of essays, spanning two centuries from 1750 to 1950, focusing on Ireland (with later chapters also incorporating Northern Ireland). It opens up for exploration the diagnosis, treatment, prevention, experience and conceptualization of childhood illness in Ireland, and in doing so provides a lens into perceptions of sick children in Ireland. It examines the role of physicians, paediatricians, parents and other caregivers; explores sites of care including outpatient institutions, hospitals, workhouses and industrial schools; and recaptures the experiences of the child patient.

Defining the age boundaries of childhood through two centuries of Irish history is not within the remit of this volume. Historians such as Cunningham, Marland and Gijswijt-Hofstra and Cooter have chosen to adopt a very broad conception of childhood from the ages of 4 to 14, while acknowledging the generality of this approach.[28] In view of the lack of historical attention hitherto directed at the history of childhood illness in Ireland, we too have chosen to adopt this framework. Some chapters also consider infants, where they appear alongside children as objects of care and treatment.

The time span chosen to examine the issue of childhood illness is necessarily broad. Exploration of eighteenth-century interactions between medicine and children traces the genealogy of paediatric care before its emergence as a fully formed medical sub-discipline. Examinations of nineteenth-century contexts encompass lesser documented medical problems in the wake of the Famine such as ophthalmia and scrofula. Other chapters reveal a dramatic expansion in the number and type of institutions that provided medical care for children and the increasing professionalization and specialization of Irish medical communities. By the twentieth century, paediatrics had emerged as a clinical specialism and paediatricians were met with several challenges including the treatment of rickets in Dublin's poorest children and the prevention and treatment of tuberculosis.

Ireland's unique socioeconomic and political climate during the period from 1750 to 1950 provides a challenging, yet valuable, backdrop to this study. During this time, Ireland underwent political union with the United Kingdom in 1801, the state of Northern Ireland was established in 1921, the Irish Free State in 1922 and the Irish Republic in 1949. The experience of child patients, and those attending them, was set against political rebellion, the introduction of a quasi-colonial administration, the ravages of famine, emigration and violent political upheaval. Despite this backdrop, religious considerations do not permeate this volume to any great degree. In fact, religion rarely emerges as a theme within the chapters that follow. The existence of political and religious tensions in areas of child health and welfare, however, has been well documented, particularly for twentieth-century Ireland.[29] Furthermore, Greta Jones and Elizabeth Malcolm have argued that Irish medicine was deeply affected by sectarian tensions.[30] The extent to which religion, sectarian divisions and especially the Catholic Church impacted on child medicine in Ireland is certainly worthy of more historical attention.

Although much of Ireland remained overwhelmingly rural, the majority of chapters here explore childhood illness in urban settings, most notably nineteenth- and twentieth-century Dublin and, to a lesser extent, twentieth-century Belfast. The populations of both Dublin and Belfast rose significantly during this era, as did the proportion of the Irish population who could be described as urbanized, many migrating to urban centres in Ireland.[31] During this era Dublin was notorious for poor housing, overcrowding and slum conditions for its poorest inhabitants, and both Dublin and Belfast were unhealthy in comparison with British cities.[32] A number of the chapters in this volume focus on diseases presented as having strong links with poverty, such as rickets or tuberculosis.[33] This volume's emphasis on the impoverished is also related to a heavy reliance on institutional records. Workhouses, voluntary hospitals, industrial schools and district asylums were designed primarily for the destitute and poor. Nonetheless, the prevalence of children of the poor within this volume says much about the socioeconomic conditions in which childhood illness and disease arose. Very few of the children in this volume received private medical provision but instead fell under the remit of charitable or state-funded initiatives. Ireland therefore provides an intricate case study for exploring questions about childhood illness and disease. This volume is not intended as an Irish equivalent to studies such as Marland and Gijswijt-Hofstra's or Cooter's but rather aims to open up for investigation the medical history of childhood illness in an Irish context.

THEMES

This volume addresses four crucial themes. These are: sites of care for sick children, child patient experiences, key actors in their treatment and, at its core, the eventual emergence of paediatrics as a discrete medical sphere. These themes intertwine in complex ways and, accordingly, overlap with one another in the chapters that follow. Important changes in medical activity underpinned all of these themes. This story is relatively well known to historians of disease and illness. In the late eighteenth and early nineteenth centuries, constitutional medicine, with its emphasis on lifestyle, diet, overall constitution and external factors such as weather, still largely dictated the physician's practice. This provided a rationale for therapeutics such as bleeding, purging and the use of diuretics, which strove to achieve a balance of the four humours.[34] In addition to formally educated medical men (physicians), surgeons were engaged in performing non-intrusive operations while apothecaries dispensed medicine and medical advice.[35] In Ireland, as elsewhere, a number of other figures including wise women, herbalists, itinerant drug peddlers and quacks also provided advice and 'cures'.[36] Self-medication and family remedies, traditionally held in receipt books, were also an important aspect of medicine during this era.[37]

Beginning in France in the late eighteenth century, the advent of modern pathological anatomy had, by the post-Napoleonic period, begun to spread to England and by the 1830s had entered the medical curriculum there.[38] The rise of pathological anatomy led to new conceptions of disease as medicine began to focus more on organs, 'specific lesions or characteristic functional changes that would, if not modified, produce lesions over time'.[39] In Dublin, basic modern scientific and institutional medical practice had also been established by the early nineteenth century and the city had begun developing into 'a major centre of medical education, on a par with London and Edinburgh'.[40] In line with the new, increasingly scientific approach to medicine, the Dublin School of Medicine had a 'coterie of famous medical men who developed a set of medical and research practices unique in the British Isles'.[41]

By the mid-nineteenth century, Dublin was host to a number of teaching hospitals, medical schools and medical colleges.[42] This period also witnessed the increasing importance of the laboratory to medical education, beginning in Germany before spreading to other western countries.[43] This new branch of medical science was characterized by laboratory investigations, rather than observations made at the patient's bedside, and ultimately rendered observable the aetiological importance of bacteria and germs to diseases of both childhood and adulthood. From the 1870s, the development of germ theories began to gain currency among the medical profession. There was a shift from understanding disease as being caused by multiple factors with a predisposing cause (e.g. poverty, dirt, bad air) towards understanding disease as being caused by a single entity observable and treatable only through medico-scientific intervention. Thus by the twentieth century the framing of disease had largely shifted from physiological to ontological models. New approaches to diagnosis, prevention and treatment therefore focused upon the recognition and removal of causes such as germs or bacteria.[44] How, then, did changes in medicine impact on the medical care of children from

1750 to 1950? To what extent did wider developments in medicine influence the sites, experiences and key overseers of childhood illness?

The sites of childhood illness and treatment certainly adjusted in line with changes in medical knowledge. Several chapters in this volume focus upon institutions where medical care and treatment was offered to children. These include voluntary children's hospitals, lock hospitals, workhouses, lunatic asylums, reformatories and industrial schools. This inherent diversity reflects broader developments in medical provision. In the eighteenth century a network of medical charities (voluntary hospitals, county infirmaries, dispensaries and fever hospitals) evolved in Ireland, providing free medical aid to the sick poor.[45] In this period hospitals were generally controlled by boards of governors or religious orders, which had the power to select patients based on the degree to which they were considered 'deserving'.[46] The extent to which children received inpatient care in these institutions is not addressed in this volume. However, writing in 1818, Irish historians J. Warburton, Reverend James Whitelaw and Reverend Robert Walsh 'claimed that hospitals were not suitable for children and "this interesting class of society" could best receive medical attention at a dispensary'.[47] They insisted on the authority of the mother, whose 'watchful anxiety can alone distinguish, for the physician's guidance, symptoms impervious to any but a mother's eye'.[48] In the British context Andrea Tanner has noted that 'poor sick children were largely excluded from wards of voluntary hospitals until the 1850s'.[49] The extent to which children received inpatient care in Irish general hospitals warrants further attention.

During the nineteenth century hospitals became centres of medical education and research, a product of the increasing application of science to medicine. Stemming from this, the first dedicated children's hospital in Ireland, the Dublin Institution for the Diseases of Children (DIDC), was founded in 1822. This hospital initially provided an outpatients service only. It was highly influential in the development of models for the management of childhood diseases and predated the establishment of children's hospitals in Britain by almost thirty years.[50] While the DIDC was funded through voluntary donations from the public, it was set up by medical professionals. However, as this volume demonstrates, accommodating children in institutions often generated anxieties. Debates centred on the provision of special wards in general hospitals, the mixing of adult and child patients and the provision of separate hospitals for children. These concerns formed part of evolving ideas about childhood and where children belonged. By the mid-nineteenth century, efforts were being made to reduce the number of children in workhouses through the establishment of district schools and the introduction of the boarding out of workhouse children, both under the Irish Poor Law.[51] However, industrial schools were established with the intention of providing accommodation for children who might otherwise succumb to criminality in the absence of a stable domestic environment.[52] Rhetoric concerning the propriety of institutionalizing children was thus contingent on a number of social factors. In terms of hospitalization, Tanner has found that the first children's hospital in Britain was met with 'considerable opposition from the medical establishment and lay opinion that decreed children were not suitable objects for hospital treatment'.[53]

In addition to growing diversity in hospital care, the centralization of government in nineteenth-century Ireland following the Act of Union generated an increase in the number, size and variety of state-sponsored institutions. In 1817 legislation was enacted to provide 'asylums for the lunatic poor'.[54] These asylums also catered for children, albeit on a very small scale.[55] Following the Famine, the Irish Poor Law was a key locus of medical provision for the poor.[56] Medical influence also extended over various institutions including workhouses, reformatories and industrial schools.[57] What emerges from the scholarship in this volume is that, similar to the piecemeal way in which Irish medical practice developed for adults, there was no single coherent network of paediatric care in Ireland for much of the period under study. Instead, nineteenth-century Irish institutions sometimes became accidental sites of medical care whose primary roles were somewhat overshadowed by the necessity to treat diseases such as scrofula or ophthalmia.[58] That several of the chapters in this book focus on institutions perhaps says as much about the availability of primary material as it does about the actuality of children's medicine during this period. For instance, more research might be directed towards the medical care and treatment of children in a domestic setting, and private medical initiatives. Nevertheless, the level of institutionalization of children until the late twentieth century has been described as one of the 'abiding features of child welfare in Ireland', and this volume suggests that this was paralleled within a healthcare framework.[59] The increasing medicalization of childhood illness was reflected in the rising number of specialized institutions for sick children in Ireland.

The extent to which medical advances impacted upon experiences of childhood illness is more difficult to quantify because the experience of the child patient is especially challenging to retrieve. In 2003 Marland and Gijswijt-Hofstra asserted that 'the history of the sick child has not advanced so far' and issued a challenge 'to find the child in the competing discourses surrounding health, and to develop a child-centred approach'.[60] Some contributors to this volume have taken up this call using oral histories, case notes and case histories. The recollections of adult survivors of childhood illness shed light on their experiences in both domestic and institutional settings. These oral histories provide a poignant account of the child patients' understanding of their illness, the role of the family, neighbours, institutions, doctors and nurses as well as the lasting consequences – both emotional and physical – on those who contracted infection. While oral histories clearly lend unique insight into the experiences of childhood illness – experiences that would otherwise go undocumented – this methodology is only possible for diseases experienced within living memory. For an earlier period, case notes and histories reveal a sense of the child patient's experiences of illness in an institutional setting, albeit mediated through the infrequent observations of medical personnel.

In addition to the experience of the child, this volume explores the wide range of actors involved in decisions pertaining to the treatment and care of sick children. Chapters in this volume demonstrate that key actors in the management of childhood illness ranged from mothers to government officials and from physicians to philanthropists. Parents' reactions to illness in a child are demonstrated in the context of the build-up to, and aftermath of, smallpox inoculation in eighteenth-century Ireland. Parental responses are also mediated through the oral histories of adult survivors of twentieth-century childhood illness. It could be argued that despite the evident changes in the conceptualization of childhood from the eighteenth to twentieth centuries, parents of Irish children apparently reacted with similar grief at the death or serious illness of their child. This supports the finding by Linda Pollock that there was no change in the extent of parental grief from the sixteenth to twentieth centuries at the death of a child, while parents in all centuries were distressed and anxious at their illness.[61] Pat Jalland, in her study of death in the Victorian family, has lent support to this thesis, stressing that 'like us, most Victorians believed that the death of a child was the most distressing and incapacitating of all'.[62]

In the eighteenth century the medical care of sick children lay quite firmly in the hands of parents, and particularly mothers.[63] In line with the rise of scientific medicine, physicians increasingly supplanted parents as children's primary healthcare providers. For much of the period under study, those providing medical care to children were more often general purveyors of medicine rather than those who specialized in children's medicine. Although clinical specialities in the modern sense emerged in Europe in the early nineteenth century, the number of specialists was small.[64] In Ireland, Dublin School of Medicine luminaries such as William Wilde, father of Oscar, also honed expertise in specific areas, in Wilde's case the eye and the ear.[65] This reflects shifts from understanding illness and disease as constitutional to understanding the roots of disease as resting in specific organs.

During this era, children also gained increasing recognition as a distinct patient category. By the 1830s, Irish physicians Richard Evanson and Henry Maunsell, who had been both students and later medical attendants at the

DIDC, clearly distinguished infants and children as a special category of patient, requiring a separate or modulated type of medical treatment different from that meted out to adults. In their seminal textbook on childhood illness they wrote:

> Most medicines act with great energy on the child, and some have a peculiarity of action differing from that on the adult; while all require to be given in diminishing doses, regulated by age.[66]

Despite this early recognition, paediatrics as a clinical specialism was slow to develop.[67] By 1900, there were only a handful of specialist paediatricians in Britain.[68] The reasons for this delayed emergence may lie in Annmarie Adams' and David Theodore's suggestion that when it did originate, it was not in connection to particular diseases or organs 'but rather in a meliorist program for the social reform of childhood'.[69] Certainly, paediatrics' rise in significance from the early twentieth century was in step with contemporary health and welfare developments aimed at improving infant welfare and national vitality. In 1904 the *British Journal of Diseases of Children* was launched, followed by the foundation of the British Paediatric Association in 1928. An Irish counterpart to this association (the Irish Paediatric Club, later the Irish Paediatric Association) was set up in 1933 and its membership boasted several prominent Irish paediatricians including Ella Webb, Dorothy Price, Kathleen Lynn and Robert Collis.[70] Its inauguration highlights the growing prominence of Irish paediatrics in this period.

Nonetheless, ten years after its foundation, Collis complained that paediatrics had 'never been regarded as a major subject in Great Britain or Ireland'.[71] Collis was a particularly active member of the paediatric profession. Having served as house physician and later research fellow at Great Ormond Street Children's Hospital in London he returned to Dublin in 1932 and was appointed as physician to the National Children's Hospital and director of the Department of Paediatrics at the Rotunda Hospital.[72]

After the Second World War, he went to Belsen, Germany and worked with child survivors of the concentration camp and had several orphans transferred to the Fairy Hill Hospital in Howth, Dublin. He adopted two of these children and later went on to found the National Cerebral Palsy Clinic in Ireland.[73] As pointed out in this volume, the increased focus on diseases such as childhood tuberculosis in Great Britain and Ireland rendered paediatricians and their work visible. The prominence of doctors such as Collis further illustrates a high degree of activity among Irish paediatricians. It was these factors that provided validity for the continuing development of paediatrics as a separate clinical specialism.

OUTLINE OF CHAPTERS

Given the centrality of the development of scientific medicine to this volume's exploration of childhood illness, chapters are arranged chronologically. This structure was adopted in order to facilitate an understanding of broader developments in medicine and changing attitudes towards the treatment and care of sick children. Gabrielle Ashford's analysis of smallpox inoculation in the eighteenth century provides a valuable starting point, invoking a number of key themes. Her chapter meditates on the role of the parent, and specifically the mother, in the provision of child healthcare during the second half of the eighteenth century. Ashford illustrates the range of emotions articulated by parents and doctors both in the build-up to and aftermath of a child's inoculation against smallpox. For Ashford, the eventual 'professionalization' of medicine had its roots in medical appropriation (by both orthodox and unorthodox practitioners) of preventive vaccination against smallpox during this era, a development that presaged the diminishing role of the parent in child medical care in later periods.

Through his study of the DIDC, professor of paediatrics and medical historian Conor Ward explores the debates that arose concerning the increasing specialization of institutional medical provision for Irish children. He provides a chronology of children's clinics, wards and hospitals established in Ireland's capital city during the nineteenth century. The older tradition of admitting children to adult wards because of fears of infection was superseded as the century progressed and children's wards and hospitals were founded. Ward demonstrates the influence of the DIDC on the development of inpatient provision for children in England. In particular he points to the influence of the textbook *A Practical Treatise on the Management and Diseases of Children* mentioned above. Ward's chapter provides a useful backdrop to the early era of medical professionalism in Ireland and explores the debates which arose concerning a tendency towards specialization in the medical care of children.

Jean Walker's chapter focuses upon another singular Dublin institution, the Westmoreland Lock Hospital, which treated syphilitic children as well as adults. The child patient in the Lock Hospital was rarely overtly acknowledged in the nineteenth century. Walker's examination of the records of the hospital and the medical literature produced by its numerous affiliates elucidates the treatment, conceptualization and stigmatization of child-sufferers of syphilis. Walker suggests that the congenitally syphilitic child's distinctive appearance and poor prognosis were framed within a discourse of moral retribution, with the 'sins of the father' or mother visited upon the offspring. However, she also points out that in mid-nineteenth-century Ireland, syphilitic children were recognized by the medical profession as a discrete patient category calling for separate treatment strategies. Although the medical profession often appeared sympathetic to this category of patient, Walker highlights the use of these children in experimental research.

Impaired vision and blindness followed an epidemic of ophthalmia among children in Irish workhouses between 1849 and 1861. Philomena Gorey's contribution to this volume provides a salutary reminder that the shadows cast by the Famine were far-reaching. According to Gorey, the generation of children who grew up in the decades following the Famine were at a physical disadvantage. For those admitted to workhouses, overcrowding and poor nutrition rendered them vulnerable to ophthalmia, a disease that could lead to blindness and that was thought to be contagious. The role of the elite medical practitioner is highlighted as the severity and persistence of the epidemic prompted the Poor Law Commissioners to call on specialist medical practitioners Arthur Jacob and William Wilde. In addition to ophthalmic expertise, Wilde brought a statistical expertise to his analysis of the disease outbreak. Gorey suggests, however, that although famine conditions emphasized the high risk and incidence of the disease, it did not affect or advance medical knowledge.

June Cooper's discussion of epilepsy (1850–1904), the only chapter to address mental illness in children, examines recommendations for the treatment of epilepsy including orthodox and non-orthodox treatments. This chapter also provides a case study of an institutional response to epileptic children by examining the records of the Richmond District Lunatic Asylum. As such, it speaks to Conor Ward's discussion of separate accommodation for children in Irish institutions in the nineteenth century. Cooper recaptures a sense, through the infrequent observations of medical personnel, of the history of a child's care and, to an extent, experiences of illness in an institutional setting. Cooper posits that the asylum proffered children better access to medical assistance than they might have received in workhouses or neglectful family homes. Nonetheless, she remarks on the sense of cessation following admission as particularly palpable in the case of children, a small number of whom grew up in the Richmond and died at Portrane.

In Ian Miller's chapter, the theme of post-Famine sequelae with respect to children explored in Gorey's chapter is revisited, albeit with a moral emphasis. Miller demonstrates that the migration of youths to the city of Dublin following the Famine was blamed for increasing levels of juvenile delinquency. Children deprived of a suitable familial environment were perceived as requiring institutionalization to guard against their potential corruption in the criminal world. Miller contends that as child criminality became increasingly interpreted as linked to abnormal bodily and mental growth, new techniques of governing bodies and minds emerged. These were embodied in the preventative and curative regimes of reformatories and industrial schools. Ian Miller provides a fresh perspective on the genesis of these institutions, demonstrating what this system of institutional childcare was initially intended to be and providing a useful reference point for understanding how these institutions later transmuted into places associated with fear and abuse.

The historiography of tuberculosis in Ireland has paid considerably more attention to the adult experience of the disease than to childhood forms of tuberculosis. In this volume Anne Mac Lellan and Susan Kelly address childhood tuberculosis from two different viewpoints. Mac Lellan's chapter discusses the use and neglect of tuberculin testing for the diagnosis of tuberculosis in Irish children in the first half of the twentieth century. The consequences of the relative neglect of this test by the Irish medical profession ranged from unnecessary enforced bedrest for prolonged periods for children wrongly diagnosed as tubercular to denial of rest and treatment for children with undiagnosed tuberculosis. She highlights the role of tuberculin testing in epidemiological studies used to map tuberculosis infection in Irish children. Mac Lellan suggests that in both Great Britain and Ireland, the increased focus on childhood tuberculosis rendered paediatricians and their work visible and provided validity for the continuing development of paediatrics as a separate clinical specialism.

Laura Kelly's analysis of Irish children with rickets who were treated in the Children's Sunshine Home from 1925 to 1946 complements the other institutional histories delineated in this volume. Her work also speaks to the discussions of ophthalmia and tuberculosis which, along with rickets, share an association with poverty and diet although rickets is not contagious. Kelly suggests that the work of Ella Webb, who founded the home, may be situated within a scheme of philanthropic social work conducted by a network of Irish women doctors in Dublin which especially focused on women and children. Dorothy Price, also mentioned in Mac Lellan's chapter, fits into this scheme. Webb was the daughter of a Church of Ireland clergyman, although the home was founded on non-sectarian lines and did not engage in proselytism.

Kelly's chapter adds to a growing body of work exploring gender and religion in the context of female Irish doctors.

Ida Milne utilizes oral histories from adult survivors of the Spanish influenza epidemic of 1818–19 in order to shed light on their childhood experiences of the illness. Milne's sample discusses children's experiences of illness within the domestic setting, providing an insight into the domestic treatment of childhood illness. Evidence of the health, social and economic impact of the disease is gleaned. Milne's interviews provide poignant accounts of the child patients' understanding of their illness, the perceived impact it had on the family unit, the role of the community in providing aid to infected families and, uniquely, the lasting consequences – both emotional and physical – on those who contracted the infection. Milne contends that the interview process can be a two-way one, with the interviewer accessing a rich source of material not otherwise available and the interviewee using the interview to make sense of a traumatic childhood experience.

Susan Kelly has also recorded oral histories, which she uses in her chapter in conjunction with personal testimonies, hospital archives, government publications and contemporary medical and nursing literature to illustrate the psychological and emotional effects of bone and joint tuberculosis on children as well as its treatment. Kelly asserts that sufferers of bone and joint tuberculosis, often children, were in hospital longer, had a more complicated response to treatment and could be left with more long-term problems than their contemporaries with pulmonary tuberculosis. Kelly's interrogation of the child patient experience differs from Milne's in that her interviewees received treatment in an institutional setting, and many discussed their interactions with fellow patients. Parents' reactions to illness in a child are also mediated through the recollections of the adult survivors in Kelly's and Milne's chapters. While oral histories provide unique insights into the experiences of childhood illness – experiences that would otherwise go undocumented – this methodology is, of course, only possible for diseases within living memory.

These chapters, taken together, do not purport to be a comprehensive history of childhood illness in Ireland. Instead they offer a starting point from which such an exploration might be undertaken. In doing so it is hoped that this volume will open up childhood illness in Ireland as a fruitful ground for exploration and that it will stimulate further research in this and other areas of Irish medical history.

1

Children's Smallpox and Inoculation Procedures in Eighteenth-Century Ireland

Gabrielle Ashford

O f all the diseases listed in eighteenth-century bills of mortality, it was
smallpox that had, by far, the most devastating impact on children's
lives. The variola virus was an indiscriminate killer, affecting children of
all social classes. It was responsible for 20 per cent of all deaths in Dublin
between 1661 and 1745[1] and for the premature deaths of one third of
children in Ireland between 1717 and 1746.[2] By international standards,
these were extremely high mortality figures. In comparison, during the
eighteenth century smallpox was responsible for the deaths of only 10 per
cent of all those born in Sweden and 14 per cent in Russia.[3] Consequently the
expansion of smallpox inoculation in Ireland had, arguably, the greatest and
most significant medical benefit to Irish society as a whole and to children
in particular.

Its manifest benefits notwithstanding, the acceptance and practice of
inoculation was not without debate, both within medicine and among
parents. For example, the correct time and season for inoculation, the

necessity for elaborate pre- and post-inoculation procedures and, indeed, the legitimacy and contagiousness of the inoculation procedure formed the basis of animated discussions, and even though the introduction of a safer and more successful technique in 1762 had the 'most amazing success',[4] not everyone was convinced. Yet as this chapter illustrates, from mid-century more and more children of all social classes in Ireland were inoculated or gained some form of immunity from the disease.

This chapter contrasts the smallpox and inoculation experiences of families from a variety of social backgrounds over the course of the eighteenth century. It advances the argument that the degree of wealth families possessed impacted significantly on the mode of treatment their children received after contracting natural smallpox, and likewise in the procedures adopted in preparation for, and during, inoculation. Moreover, it contends that the unprecedented degree of medical intervention in children's healthcare instigated by inoculation procedures was important to the 'professionalization' of medical practice in eighteenth-century Ireland. Although parents, especially mothers, continued to take a dominant role in the medical supervision of their sick children in eighteenth-century Ireland, the control exercised by physicians during the course of inoculation established a new trend, and presaged the diminishing role that parents were to assume in the medical care of children in later periods.[5] The fact that the debates surrounding smallpox inoculation occurred in tandem with the growing acceptance of the idea that the child, as an individual, required specific care and attention discrete from the adult, helped to reinforce the emerging concept of childhood that was a distinctive feature of the eighteenth century.[6]

CHILDREN'S MEDICAL CARE IN EIGHTEENTH-CENTURY IRELAND

Although children's health was a major preoccupation for parents in eighteenth-century Ireland, there was no comprehensive medical network in the country, and with the exception of the Lying-In Hospital (1745) children were largely excluded from institutional medical care facilities. Accordingly families faced formidable health challenges when negotiating childhood. On the one hand, parents were acutely aware of the fallibility of available medicines and medical advice, while on the other hand, physicians were 'prepared to take few risks like using unknown potions',[7] especially in relation to children.

At the beginning of the eighteenth century an absence of publications relating to childhood healthcare ensured that parents did not have access to information in print to assess and treat their children's ills. Moreover, a lack of comprehensive medical facilities – indeed, in some cases of any at all – obliged parents, but generally women, to resort to a variety of strategies – medical and otherwise – in response. Mothers were expected to be self-reliant and to take the primary role in alleviating family illnesses. Within elite and gentry families, this sustained the maintenance of the domestic medical receipt book and obliged recourse to self-diagnosis and self-medication.[8] When children were sick or ailing, mothers, in the first instance, looked for guidance to their domestic receipt books, and for advice and counsel to their family and friends. In Ireland as in Britain, family domestic receipt books were highly valued, and the fact that they were handed down through the generations indicates their importance. But more important is the fact that women updated, commented on and continued to collect receipts into the nineteenth century.

Mirroring an ongoing debate among medical authorities about the merits of self-diagnosing, by the 1770s parental opinion regarding children's medicines and parental attitudes towards medical intervention diverged. Although proprietary medicines targeted specifically at children, such as *Bennet's Worm Cakes*, became more widely available towards the end of the eighteenth century,[9] women continued to accumulate domestic receipts to assist them in administering to their children. These facts highlight three important points: in the first instance, the fallibility of the medical advice and medicines given throughout the eighteenth century; secondly, the crucial role women played in the domestic medical care of children during the eighteenth century; and thirdly, that in the case of children the patient's authority lay firmly and emphatically in the hands of the parent, and overwhelmingly with mothers. Though this situation largely remained unchanged until the nineteenth century, the mid-century embrace of smallpox inoculation is significant in that it foreshadowed the passage of control from the parent/patient to the medical practitioner.

SMALLPOX EPIDEMICS IN EIGHTEENTH-CENTURY IRELAND

Smallpox epidemics swept across Ireland with alarming regularity throughout the eighteenth century.[10] A 1708 epidemic was noted as being of the 'most crude and worst kind that swept away multitudes'.[11] An epidemic of 1728 began in early winter and abated in spring. But as the winter advanced, so did the numbers of people infected, and the severity of their symptoms.[12] Exacerbated by looming famine conditions, smallpox spread throughout Ireland in May 1740 and increased to epidemic proportions over the summer. The Dublin Quaker and physician John Rutty (1697–1775) ascribed blame to beggars' children 'full of the smallpox [who] were frequently exposed' in the streets.[13] The speed with which the disease spread and claimed its victims was correspondingly alarming. Rutty recorded sixteen deaths in Cork in one week of July 1740; by August it had risen to twenty-two and then to thirty-three per week.[14] By September 1745, an average of twenty-four people per week had died from the disease, with deaths exceeding recoveries.[15] According to the Dublin Huguenot Meliora Adlercron, the smallpox outbreak in Dublin of September 1766 was 'of so virulent a nature that nineteen out of twenty [children] died of it'; she was thankful for the safe recovery of her son John and daughter Elizabeth, which she attributed to the attendance of not one but two doctors during their illness.[16]

DEVELOPMENT OF INOCULATION PROCEDURES

Inoculation was the only certain method of ensuring that children would avoid the ravages of smallpox. Introduced into Ireland at the beginning of the eighteenth century, from mid-century onwards it became more widely accepted and practised, and remained popular until superseded by the safer cow-pock vaccine at the beginning of the nineteenth century. Inoculation or variolation involved the artificial infection of healthy subjects with smallpox in the hope of producing a mild case of the disease and subsequent immunity.

Having witnessed the benefits of 'engrafting' (inoculating) against smallpox, then routinely carried out in Turkish towns and villages, Lady Mary Wortley Montagu (1689–1762), wife of the British ambassador to Turkey at the beginning of the eighteenth century, helped to promote and popularize the system of inoculation on her return to England. Adopted first by the elite, it quickly filtered down the social order, dovetailing on occasions with existing precautionary procedures. In 1722 Richard Wright, a surgeon at Haverford West, Wales, recorded a longstanding tradition among the population in that area of 'buying the small pox' in order to provide protection.[17] He noted that the inhabitants of the villages of St Ishmael's and Marloes near Milford Haven, Pembrokeshire were particularly renowned for the practice, which was recorded as occurring as early as the 1630s.[18] However, this tradition remained local.

There were crucial differences in the inoculation methods practised in Turkey and England. From the start of inoculation in England, the medical profession used a lancet to make a deep cut in the flesh. Scraping the skin's surface to receive the virus in the manner employed in Turkey was a more efficacious method and had better results. The critical importance of the depth of the incision was not recognized by English physicians, so by employing the English lancet method the success rate of children's early inoculation was significantly reduced.[19]

Emanuel Timoni and Giacomo Pylarini (1659–1718) are credited with publishing, in England, the first medical accounts of their inoculation procedures in 1713 and 1715 respectively.[20] Dublin physician Bryan Robinson compiled the first published report in Ireland of inoculating children against smallpox a decade later in August 1725.[21] Compared with the noted Swiss physician Samuel-Auguste Tissot's (1728–1797) later 1766 calculation of

14 per cent mortality, Robinson's early inoculation practices recorded a discouraging 50 per cent mortality rate.[22] Other contemporary accounts confirm that early inoculation procedures were unreliable and remained so until mid-century.

ATTITUDES AND RESPONSES TO INOCULATION

Parental doubt surrounding smallpox and inoculation is manifest in Irish eighteenth-century correspondence and in contemporary medical books. Despite the attendant risk, the dangers of smallpox encouraged an increasing number of parents to try inoculation. Though seized with anxiety both before and after the event, Mrs Forth Hamilton, a friend of the artist and letter writer Mary Delany (1700–88) of Delville, had her two children inoculated in May 1747.[23]

As in Scotland and England, frequent outbreaks of smallpox, especially during the second and third quarters of the eighteenth century, drove some philanthropists and charitable organizations to initiate systems of mass inoculation among poor children, although these Irish schemes were never as extensive as those carried out in English cities such as Chester in 1778.[24] The Bishop of Down, John Ryder (1743–52) was extremely satisfied with the commitment to inoculation in his diocese in 1734, claiming that it was so firmly established that 'nobody who can bear the expense of it neglects inoculating [children] after two years old'.[25]

There was, however, a distinct difference between urban attitudes to smallpox and the consequences of smallpox epidemics for rural communities. Frequent outbreaks of smallpox in urban areas fostered a more fatalistic attitude towards its arrival and impact. But while children in more isolated and smaller rural districts were relatively protected from the frequent epidemics that swept urban areas, when smallpox did strike their communities, infection and mortality rates were severe. Nonetheless, contemporary accounts indicate that when available, inoculation was widely practised in rural areas.[26] During his tour of Ireland in 1796/7 the French traveller De Latocnaye encountered an itinerant inoculator in

County Mayo who had 'taken some lessons in the hospitals' and had, he claimed, been practising his craft among the Irish peasantry for thirty or forty years.[27]

Smallpox was no respecter of social status and all children were susceptible. According to influential Scottish medical doctor William Buchan (1729–1805) it was common among the poor and especially in institutions. Moreover, its spread within institutions was accelerated by poor medical practice; Buchan noted that it was not unusual for two or three children suffering from smallpox to lie in the same bed 'with such a load of pustules that even their skins stick together'.[28] Institutional governors, however, took steps to limit the spread of the disease among children in their care. Perhaps acknowledging the contagious nature of smallpox, the governors of the Dublin House of Industry (established 1773) instructed their medical officers in December 1782 to remove children suffering from smallpox to a distant house, furnished as an infirmary where they could be given medical attention.[29] There is, however, no record to suggest that they attempted to inoculate the children in their care. This may have been because there were fewer children in the care of the House of Industry overall and, crucially, many of those were of an age to have already gained immunity.

The Dublin Workhouse and Foundling Hospital (established 1703 and 1729), which dealt with greater numbers of and younger children, did attempt to inoculate those admitted to its care, although, it must be noted, unenthusiastically. As Figures 1 and 2 illustrate, between 1789 and 1796, of the 3,913 children admitted to the hospital only 12 per cent (463) were inoculated against smallpox yet 92 per cent (3,615) were listed as 'cured' of the disease. It is notable that only 8 per cent (298) died from smallpox.

Given the crowded conditions in which Foundling Hospital children lived, coupled with congestion in the infirmary, it is likely that the large number of children listed as 'cured' either obtained a mild form of the disease or an immunity that protected them.[30] In addition, most infants admitted to the hospital were discharged after short periods to be cared for by country

Figure 1. Children inoculated in the Dublin Workhouse and Foundling Hospital, 1789-96.

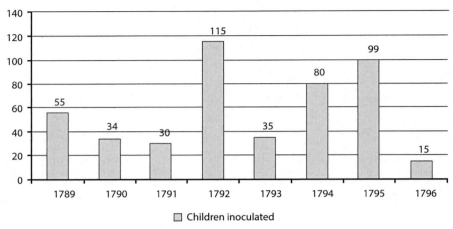

Source: *Commons Jn. (Irl.)*, 1797, vol. 17, appendix cclxxiv.

Figure 2. Number of Admissions and Outcome of Children's Smallpox and Inoculation in the Dublin Workhouse and Foundling Hospital, 1789-96.

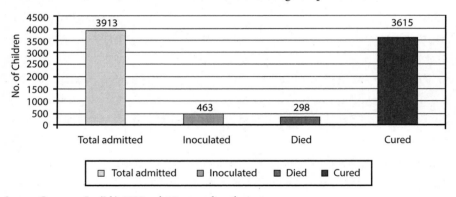

Source: *Commons Jn. (Irl.)*, 1797, vol. 17, appendix cclxxiv.

nurses, and only returned to the hospital at the age of six. Consequently they may already have established immunity to smallpox. In practice, smallpox did not reach epidemic proportions in Irish eighteenth-century institutions.

DEBATES SURROUNDING INOCULATION PROCEDURES AND PRACTICES

Early reports of smallpox inoculation procedures and practices were the subject of much discussion and debate throughout the eighteenth century. The type of pox (benign or confluent), the patient's age and sex, preparing the child, and indeed the exact method of inoculation were all matters of active debate. The Cork-based physician Joseph Rogers (1677–1753) directed that the 'pock', of the most 'benign' sort, be taken from an otherwise healthy child younger than 7 years old, laid on a piece of lint and inserted using a lancet in the arm and leg only.[31] On the seventh day after inoculation the symptoms would appear. The fact that Rogers specifically warned against making 'too many incisions' suggests that it was a common practice among inoculators to make multiple incisions on the body. By 1769 renowned physician William Buchan advised parents to inoculate children themselves using a safer, more reliable, method than Rogers'.

Choosing the most apt season in which to inoculate was problematic. Buchan considered the beginning of winter the best time, followed by spring or autumn. England-based inoculation pioneer Thomas Dimsdale (1712–1800), writing in 1774, disagreed. He recommended that inoculation be carried out in all seasons. Complicating the issue further, others claimed that the severity of smallpox was dependent on the patient's age and sex. While humoral medicine decreed that women's and children's bodies were more susceptible to the disease because of their 'moist' natures, they were also seen as being more capable of enduring its effects.[32] Young men 'in the flower of [their] age', however, were perceived to be at greater risk from the impacts of smallpox.[33] Tissot also recognized children's different constitutions – robust or weak – and its implication for inoculation,[34] whereas the Swedish physician and founder of modern 'paediatrics' Nils Rosén von Rosenstein (1706–73) attached importance not only to the child's constitution but also their lifestyle, suggesting that the latter influenced the severity of the resultant smallpox.[35]

The age at which a child was inoculated was also thought to determine the outcome. Rogers claimed to have successfully inoculated his own child at 7 months old *circa* 1710,[36] whereas Buchan at mid-century recommended inoculating children between 3 and 5 years of age. Doing so sooner could lead to what he described as 'many disagreeable circumstances'.[37] Dimsdale also recommended that children under 2 years of age should not be inoculated.[38] Von Rosenstein, however, offered a choice, from 4 to 14 and from 16 to 25 years of age.[39]

Given the high mortality rate among children from smallpox, visible confirmation of a successful inoculation was not an unreasonable demand and was the subject of active debate among physicians. Generally, the outbreak of approximately one hundred spots was deemed confirmation. Anne Cooke (1726–1809) kept a record over seventeen days of the progress of her children's inoculation pocks.[40] Despite her doctor's reassurance, a concerned Lady Louisa Conolly (1743–1821) remarked in 1786 that she would 'have been much better satisfied if [her foster-daughter Emmy] had had a few spots'.[41] An anxious Marianne Fortescue (1767–1849) of Drumcar, County Louth had her daughter Emily (1797–1860) inoculated in 1799, even though she thought 'she had it before'.[42]

These debates and differences of opinion compounded the uncertainties of parents who sought to protect their children from the ravages of smallpox. Discouraging success rates of early inoculation practices were of concern. So too was a lack of clear medical consensus on which parents could base their decisions on when best to inoculate their children and at what age, as well as to gauge its success.

INTRODUCTION OF THE SUTTONIAN METHOD OF INOCULATION

The implementation of the safer and more successful Suttonian technique in England circa 1762[43] further heightened the debate. Though still using a lancet, Robert Sutton's method of inoculation was more in line with the original Turkish practice of scraping the epidermis rather than making a deep incision. In order to promote their method in Ireland, the Sutton family's Irish agent Robert Houlton published a pamphlet in Dublin in 1768[44] in which he outlined the advantages of the Suttonian method over others. It is also fair to say that the pamphlet's publication drew welcome publicity for Sutton's recently appointed Irish agents who shrewdly based their practices in more populous and therefore more financially lucrative areas (Figure 3).

Though doubts persisted, Sutton's innovation not only significantly reduced the severity of the child's symptoms but was also manifestly more successful than other procedures. Consequently, the numbers of children inoculated by this method rose dramatically from mid-century. By 1786 Betsy Sheridan (1758–1837), sister of the Irish playwright Richard Brinsley Sheridan (1751–1816), considered that with 'proper care', the dangers of inoculation in a healthy child were 'now almost less than a common cold'.[45]

Figure 3. Agents appointed by the Sutton Family to 'regulate and extend their Art over the Kingdom of Ireland'.

Messrs Houlton, Blake & Sparrow, Surgeons, Dublin.

John Harley, MD, Cork.

John Morgan, MD, Strabane, Tyrone.

John M'Donell, MD, Cashel, Tipperary.

[Name torn] Belfast, Antrim.

Peter M'Kiough/M'Keogh, MD, Galway.

Francis Gervais, Surgeon, Naas, Athy, Co. Kildare.

Richard Doherty, Surgeon, Carlow.

Messrs Vachell & Ward Surgeons, soon to be appointed to particular districts in Ireland.

Source: Robert Houlton, *Indisputable Facts relative to the Suttonian art of Inoculation: with Observations on its Discovery, Progress, Encouragement, Opposition* (Dublin: W. G. Jones, 1768).

Nathanial Cooper's wife was so satisfied with the inoculation of her daughter in 1796 that she went 'to a play in Drogheda' that night.[46] For Limerick Methodist Elizabeth Bennis, however, the inoculation of her children in 1760 'out of obedience to [her] husband' prompted a deep religious conflict.[47] Although the issue of predestination and children's inoculation was strongly debated in Scotland (especially among islanders) and parts of England, Elizabeth Bennis apart, it does not generally appear to have been a matter of particular concern to Irish parents.

INOCULATION PROCESSES AND PROCEDURES

The disagreements and debates surrounding the best season, age and inoculation method and procedure to be used served to weaken elite and gentry parents' confidence in their capacity to decide upon the most appropriate medical care for their children. Physicians fully exploited this situation. Indicative of the emerging professionalization of medical practice, in Ireland as in England, physicians unnecessarily controlled the inoculation preparation procedures (which remained unchanged until the close of the century) and the process itself. This, of course, was financially advantageous for the physician. While elite and gentry families with the financial means to access such services did so, the costs involved effectively excluded the poor, who continued to rely on travelling inoculators and philanthropic ventures.

Humoral theory dictated that the body should be receptive to the inoculation virus and, accordingly, elaborate preparations supervised by the physician were required for two or three weeks before inoculation.[48] Elite children took up residence in the physician's home while those of the gentry or middling sort were visited by a physician daily. The blood was first cleansed for receipt of the virus. A low (vegetarian) diet, purging, bleeding and low living were seen as absolutely necessary. During the smallpox epidemics of 1718–21, Rogers commenced the inoculation procedure by bleeding, followed by the administration of a vomit and then a purge, the staple eighteenth-century medical routine.[49] Although under constant medical supervision, it is possible that this long preparation process, by weakening the child's constitution, also exposed them to the possibility of contracting smallpox naturally, particularly those residing in a physician's house for the duration of the procedure.

Once inoculated, children were kept 'cool', given a light diet such as panada or 'bread boiled with equal quantities of milk and water, good apples, roasted or boiled with milk, and sweetened with a little sugar, or such like'.[50] Preferred drinks were watered milk, clear sweet whey, barley water or thin gruel, and when the pox was fully out, buttermilk, considered of a 'cleansing nature', could be substituted.[51]

The incubation period following inoculation lasted *circa* twelve days.[52] Children tended to look a little dull, listless and drowsy before symptoms showed, experienced thirst, had little appetite and were apt to sweat when taking exercise. When inoculating his son at seven months old in 1721, Rogers administered blisters on the second day of sickening and kept them constantly running for seventeen days. Although he made no comment on the child's reaction, it must have been quite distressing as he records that he applied two, three, four and sometimes five blisters at a time.[53] As the inoculation virus took effect, the child began to suffer slight fits of heat and cold that became more violent 'as the time of the eruption' approached, accompanied with pains in the head and loins, vomiting and restlessness. The pocks, resembling flea bites, appeared on the face, arms and breast about the third or fourth day from the time of sickening.[54] The child was now in the full grip of the disease and parents and physicians commenced their anxious vigil, noting each symptom as it came, and their relief as it passed.

In contrast to the elaborate inoculation procedures imposed on elite and gentry children, according to De Latocnaye peasant children behaved just as they had before the inoculation, running about and amusing themselves nearly naked. The inoculator was called to see them only when the fever took effect, administering 'a few simple remedies' to relieve the symptoms.[55] If done correctly, the result of inoculation was a mild infection and the mortality around 3 to 4 per cent.[56] Of the 361 children De Latocnaye's itinerant inoculator had inoculated that year (1796/7), he claimed that only one child had died.[57] Although the Bishop of Down, John Ryder, also boasted that of the more than one thousand children inoculated in his diocese between 1740 and 1743 only one had died,[58] low mortality was not the invariable result of inoculation campaigns. As James Kelly notes, itinerant inoculations were not always successful. Of fifty-two children inoculated in County Donegal in 1781, fifty-one died.[59] Despite the enthusiasm for inoculation among the poor, however, there were continuing but sporadic outbreaks of smallpox, although it must be said that Irish infection rates were lower than those of England and Wales.[60]

The death of a child was a constant worry for those providing medical attendance during the eighteenth century, and this was particularly so following inoculation. Remarking on the death of a friend's child subsequent to inoculation, Lady Sarah Lennox (1745–1826) observed that the mother's grief was compounded by the fact that she had the child inoculated against the father's wishes.[61] Believing he had done all that was necessary when treating the child of Lieutenant Colonel William Browne in 1783 for 'natural smallpox', Irish physician William Drennan (1745–1820) observed that 'even if the child should die I do not think that I shall lose that degree of confidence which I may have acquired'.[62] This was not always the case; De Latocnaye's itinerant inoculator faced physical retribution from grieving parents and relations. Not only was he unlikely to receive his fee, he chose to make a quick escape 'to avoid a beating by the afflicted parents'.[63]

BENEFITS OF INOCULATION

There were two significant and long-lasting after-effects for natural smallpox survivors: scarring (particularly on the face) and, among males, reduced fertility.[64] Following the uptake of inoculation, the latter no longer occurred, leading (particularly from mid-century) to a reduction in male infertility in Ireland. Arthur Young (1741–1820), the English agriculturalist and economist, observed in 1776 that the numbers of children in Fortland, Easkey, County Sligo seemed to have increased 'particularly since inoculation was introduced, which was about ten years ago'.[65] This growth may be attributable to increased male fertility and/or a reduction in child mortality. Either way, it serves to illustrate two important consequences of inoculation for eighteenth-century Irish society and its demographic history.

Scarring as a result of smallpox, which marked between 65 and 80 per cent of those affected,[66] could have devastating effects on children and particularly girls, but for many parents this was secondary to the child's survival. The impact of facial scarring on females as a result of smallpox was succinctly verbalized by Oliver Goldsmith (1730–74), the Anglo-Irish writer and poet, in 1765 when he wrote:

> Lo, the smallpox with horrid glare
> Levelled its terrors at the fair;
> And, rifling every youthful grace,
> Left but the remnant of a face.[67]

When Colonel Browne's daughter was recovering from smallpox in 1783 it was joyously reported that 'not a scar [would] remain to deface her beauty'.[68] According to William Drennan, who was in attendance throughout her illness, while her mother[69] deemed the potential facial scarring to be 'among the first of considerations', her father wished only for her life.[70] The gay, pretty, good-humoured Letty Bushe was not so lucky. Her marriage prospects suddenly diminished once she contracted natural smallpox. According to her friend Mary Delany, 'all the men were dying whilst she was in danger', but the deep facial scarring left by smallpox 'divested [her] of those charms that occasioned their devotion'.[71] Conversely, Lady Louisa Conolly commented that rather than spoiling 15-year-old Lord Edward Fitzgerald's (1763–98) face, 'being pitted' from a smallpox inoculation would rather become him.[72]

Given their otherwise weighty reliance on their domestic and medical receipt books, it is interesting to note that only a few Irish receipt books contained specific recipes for the treatment or alleviation of smallpox, natural or prophylactic. This may be because those who kept receipt books were of the elite and gentry classes and were therefore able to afford the physician's fee should their children contract smallpox. Moreover, in tandem with an increased recognition of childhood as a distinct life phase, by mid-century there was a growing number of medical authors specifically addressing the diagnosis, prognosis and treatment of children's ailments, including smallpox and inoculation. As part of the Anglophone world, Ireland had access to its books, though these were only available to those who could read and afford their cost. But it is a measure of their appeal that by the mid-eighteenth century, medical works concerning child rearing and children's healthcare originating across Europe were increasingly published in Dublin (Figure 4).[73]

Given the mid-century development of the safer and more successful Suttonian method of inoculation, and the emergence of a significant body of publications addressing the topic, parents may have felt little need to

Figure 4. Selected Dublin Publications relative to Children's Healthcare in Eighteenth-Century Ireland.

John Locke, *Some Thoughts Concerning Education* (1693) printed in Dublin in the 9th ed., 1728 twice; the 10th ed., in 1737; in 1738 and as the 15th ed., in 1778 and others.

James Nelson, *An Essay on the Government of Children* (London, 1756) reprinted in Dublin in 1763 and 1764.

Theophilus Lobb, *The Good Samaritan* (London, 1761) reprinted in Dublin in 1764.

William Buchan, *Domestic Medicine* (London, 1769) printed in Dublin in the 2nd ed., 1773; 3rd ed., 1774; 6th ed., 1777.

Samuel Tissot, *Advice to People in General* (Lyons, 1766) translated and printed in Dublin in 1766, 1769 and 1774.

William Cadogan, *An Essay upon Nursing and the Management of Children* (9th ed., Dublin, 1771).

accumulate domestic receipts to assist them in dealing with children's smallpox, natural or prophylactic. Therefore, the treatment of children's smallpox and inoculation is the one area where eighteenth-century parents bowed completely to the physician's guidance, control and advice. This changing attitude among elite and gentry Irish parents was fully exploited by physicians and forms a fundamental part of what Ginnie Smith describes as the 'professionalization of medicine'.[74]

By the end of the eighteenth century the safer 'vaccination' system developed by Dr Edward Jenner (1749–1823) that made use of a cowpox fluid had become standard.[75] The first vaccination centre in Dublin, using Jenner's method, was opened at the Dispensary for the Infant Poor at Exchequer Street in 1800. Between that date and 1806, more than 11,000 children were vaccinated.[76] Uptake among the urban poor was so great that the Cow-Pock Institution was established at North Cope Street in 1804. Children who attended the institution on Tuesdays and Saturdays between two and three o'clock were vaccinated.

CONCLUSIONS

During the eighteenth century, the medical care of children and the treatment of their diseases lay firmly within the domestic sphere. As a result parents, and especially mothers, played the dominant role in the provision of children's healthcare and a vicariously influential role in the development of 'paediatric' medical care.[77] They adopted strategies to keep their children healthy: they diagnosed, prepared and dispensed medicines in the home to their sick children; they controlled access to the sickroom (a predominantly female domain); and, though the evidence is more ambiguous on this point, they shaped the child's doctor-patient relationship. But they experienced a significant challenge to their medical authority with the introduction of smallpox inoculation.

Smallpox inoculation had considerable immediate and far-reaching consequences for society as a whole and children in particular. It not only reduced male infertility, especially from the 1760s, but it also significantly reduced child mortality. As William Bynum has noted, during the eighteenth century 'health mattered and people were prepared to pay for it'.[78] This is particularly manifest in the elaborate inoculation preparations promoted by physicians and engaged in by elite and gentry families. Yet inoculation initiatives carried out among children in Ireland's scattered and rural communities by itinerant inoculators and philanthropists were also warmly supported, and the enthusiasm with which peasant parents availed of them for their children paved the way, albeit slowly, for the absorption of such families into the Irish medical model.

Even though there was no scientific understanding of the smallpox virus during the eighteenth century on a par with our modern-day knowledge, empirically inoculation worked. The newness of inoculation procedures meant Irish parents had no store of knowledge or experience to fall back on. As a result, smallpox and inoculation is the one area of childhood medicine in eighteenth-century Ireland where parents submitted their children to the total control of the attending physician or itinerant inoculator.

Reflecting the serious implications of smallpox for all classes of society, John Russell, sixth Duke of Bedford (1766–1839), writing to William Wyndham Grenville, first Baron Grenville (1759–1834) in 1806, argued for 'compulsory measures' and 'legislative interference' to assist in the extermination of smallpox.[79] However, compulsory smallpox vaccination was not introduced in Ireland until 1863. Prior to that, from 1840 to 1862 legislation provided for free rather than compulsory vaccination.[80] This compulsory and, it must be noted, safer smallpox vaccination system had the effect of finally turning the rural poor away from itinerant smallpox inoculators to whom they had previously remained firmly committed.[81]

2

CHILDREN'S HOSPITAL SERVICES IN VICTORIAN DUBLIN: THE ROLE OF THE INSTITUTION FOR THE DISEASES OF CHILDREN (1822–1886)[1]

Conor Ward

*W*atson's *Gentleman's and Citizen's Almanack*, published in 1826, has the following entry:

> Dublin Institution for the Diseases of Children (founded 1822). No. 9 Pitt St. Patron: the Lord Lieutenant, Viscount Lorton. In this institution the Poor receive Advice and Medicine gratis, between 11 and 12 o'clock daily. Since it opened, upwards of 7,000 children have been relieved. It depends for its support on Voluntary Contributions. It is open for the instruction of Pupils, and in winter, Lectures are delivered on the Diseases of Children. Physicians: Dr Crampton, Dr Marsh and Dr Cuming. Surgeons: Phil. Crampton, Chas. Johnson, and D.B. Tarleton Esqrs. Apothecary: Mr Montgomery Ferguson. Contributions will be received by Messrs. J.D. La Touche and Company.

Treasurers: Dr Cuming, 41 Marlborough St. Secretary: Mr W.G. Hulbert, Collector, 68 Bride Street.[2]

The first provision of a specific paediatric service for children in Dublin city was through the Dublin Institution for the Diseases of Children, which was founded in 1822. Social conditions in the city were poor throughout the nineteenth century.[3] The Act of Union had resulted in the mass emigration of the wealthier classes from Dublin, and this deprived artisans of their regular living.[4] From 1822, intermittent recurrence of famine conditions led to fresh influxes of destitute farming families seeking refuge in an already overcrowded city. The pattern repeated itself many times and reached its climax at the time of the Great Famine between 1845 and 1851/2.[5]

No official statistics on infant mortality were available until 1864 when William Donnelly (1844–76), the first Registrar General in Ireland, reported that 20 per cent of newborn infants died before their first birthday.[6] Adverse conditions continued throughout the nineteenth century. Donnelly's successor Thomas Wrigley Grimshaw (1839–1900) reported in 1885 that almost 50 per cent of the population of Dublin city still lived in slum tenements in which up to eight families shared a single 'old, degenerated, dilapidated building', described as 'fourth class'. Sharing a single privy compounded the spread of infection, and 30 per cent of child deaths were due to epidemic diseases.[7] Dietary deprivation was universal among the poor. In 1833 Speer wrote that 'the diet of these poor people appears no less to predispose to disease. Potatoes are the only healthy and nutritious article employed; fresh meat, garden vegetables, milk, oatmeal, or combinations of these, may be termed luxuries with them.'[8] Similar conditions affected children in other large cities.[9]

Only two thirds of the deaths were medically certified, suggesting that one third of the children had died without receiving medical attention of any kind. Fifty per cent of families had no ascertainable income, and those children under the age of five years, driven by destitution into the workhouses, suffered a death rate of 117 per 1,000, almost seven times the death rate in the children of the professional and financially independent classes. Ten per cent died from malnutrition. Malnutrition, by impairing resistance, must have contributed greatly to the high death rate from infection.

An incredibly high 16 per cent of infant deaths were due to convulsions. The most likely explanation for this was a high incidence of rickets leading to lowering of serum calcium to a level at which convulsions might develop. Children from the tenements were at risk of getting rickets both from lack of ultraviolet light and from low dietary vitamin D intake. This problem was widespread in other cities, as noted by Rendle Short in England and by Shanks in Scotland. Rickets is still a common cause of up to 60 per cent of afebrile convulsions in countries abroad today in which social conditions mimic those of Victorian Dublin. [10] The unduly high incidence of convulsions in England and Wales continued up to the end of the nineteenth century.[11] Despite the identification of vitamin D deficiency as the underlying cause of rickets, Saunders reported as late as 1933 that it was unusual to find any Dublin child between the ages of one and two without some evidence of old or active rickets. He had good results treating idiopathic convulsions empirically with calcium and vitamin D.[12]

In Dublin's tenements skimmed milk and buttermilk were used as milk substitutes. Both are grossly deficient in vitamin D. When families could buy milk, the vitamin D content of the milk of city stall-fed cattle was predictably very low.[13] For children whose parents could not afford whole milk, the use of skimmed milk or buttermilk, both low in vitamin D, was also a possible contributory source of deficiency. Similarly serious vitamin A deficiency was common.[14]

With an infant mortality rate of 184 per 1,000 live births in the ten years from 1879 to 1888 reported by Grimshaw, conditions in Dublin clearly remained worse than in the other Irish cities.[15] In Belfast the infant mortality rate was 149 per 1,000 and in Cork it was 121 per 1,000. Dublin's problems were worse than those of the English industrial cities, where the highest mortalities were 180 per 1,000 in Liverpool, 177 per 1,000 in Manchester, 171 per 1,000 in Leeds and 162 per 1,000 in Bradford, in all of which children's mothers worked in the industrial mills.[16] Dublin's manufacturing capacity was in the doldrums following the Act of Union and there was no factory work for women, differing in this respect from English industrial cities in which working women could contribute to family income.[17]

FOUNDATION OF THE INSTITUTION FOR THE DISEASES OF CHILDREN

The Institution was set up by Henry Marsh (1790–1860), with the support of Charles Johnson (1795–1866) and John Crampton (1768–1840). Henry Marsh was later knighted, as was Philip Crampton, one of the first surgeons listed above.[18] Henry Marsh was appointed Professor of Medicine in Park Street Medical School in 1832 and Physician in Ordinary to the Queen in 1837. He was physician to Dr Steevens' Hospital. His memorial statue is on permanent exhibition in the Royal College of Physicians. Charles Johnson was an obstetrician and ex-master of the Rotunda Hospital.[19] He provided the first accommodation for the Institution in the mews of his residence in Molesworth Street. In 1822 the Institution's address was 9 Pitt Street (now Balfe Street). Pitt Street was an unfashionable address. Street directories list local residents' occupations as lower middle class. Although Henry Marsh was the son of a clergyman, he belonged to a Walkerite sect.[20] This may have been the reason that, during his lifetime, the Institution was never listed as a beneficiary of the Hospital Sunday Fund church collection organized by the Church of Ireland. It came to participate later. The Institution was an independent charity and it served the families living in the Liberties, the most deprived area in Dublin city.

John Crampton, the other founding physician, was not related to Sir Philip. He was one of the most distinguished physicians of his day. He was an MD of Edinburgh University having presented his thesis in Latin, entitled *De Amaurosi* (On Blind Persons). A Fellow of the King's and Queen's College of Physicians from 1798, he was first assistant physician to Dr Steevens' Hospital where he lectured from 1800, becoming King's Professor of Materia Medica in 1804. He was appointed physician to the Hardwicke Hospital in 1817 and it was here that he identified a boy with cyanotic congenital heart disease whose clinical signs and subsequent autopsy revealed him to be one of the earliest cases of what came to be known as the tetralogy of Fallot, but who, in addition, presented with a unique subdivision of the right ventricle. On this basis Crampton should be entitled to eponymity.[21]

This observation brought Crampton to the fore in the academic world. He was invited to write a chapter on cyanosis in the *London Encyclopaedia of Medicine*[22] and he was quoted in Bentley Todd's *Cyclopedia of Anatomy and Physiology*.[23] He was the most frequent contributor to the Transactions of the Fellows and Licentiates of the Royal College. His publication escaped the attention of Fallot but was referred to by Thomas Peacock of London, who called him 'my friend Mr Crampton'.[24] Peacock's description of the tetralogy had been published twenty years before Fallot's publication on the disorder. The paper also attracted attention in the United States and in particular it was quoted by James Stewart in 1845.[25]

Thomas Cuming, the assistant physician, also had a distinguished career. As a young man he had volunteered to attend fever patients in Richmond General Penitentiary without remuneration, his actual appointment being to the Whitworth Hospital. In the course of the year he had attended to fifty patients and he himself contracted a fever on four occasions. His 1822 description of the pulse in aortic incompetence was recognized posthumously by the eminent British cardiologist Bedford Evans.[26] Cuming also achieved national and international recognition for his observations on *cancrum oris*, a life-threatening gangrenous ulceration of the mouth. In his opinion this only occurred in the presence of severe malnutrition.[27] The paper was noted in the US by Holes and in the UK by Elliotson.[28] Cuming developed an extensive practice in his native Armagh.

THE INSTITUTION'S MEDICAL AUTHORS

In 1836 a new textbook appeared with the title *A Practical Treatise on the Management and Diseases of Children*.[29] The authors were Richard Evanson (1800–71) and Henry Maunsell (1806–79). They wrote that they had both been connected with the Institution since its establishment, first as students and subsequently as staff members. The book became very popular, and when the fifth edition was published in 1848 a preliminary chapter was added, which the authors hoped would be useful to lay people. In their preface the authors gave as the reason for publishing the book their publisher's recognition that a concise practical work on the management of diseases of children would meet a clinical need.

Two German editions and one French edition had already appeared. They identified Henry Marsh as the founder of the Institution and they dedicated the book to him as a mark of respect for his high station in the medical profession and in gratitude for many personal favours. The second and fifth editions were published in the United States with an additional chapter by David Francis Condie. A review in the *Edinburgh Medical and Surgical Journal* in 1838 was very complimentary and ranked the textbook with the authoritative works of George Armstrong, John Clark and George Underwood.[30] The book was clearly written from a background of wide clinical experience. Sound advice was given, with appropriate emphasis on breastfeeding and on the safe use of cow's milk when breastfeeding failed. The benefits of fresh air and sunshine were emphasized and the clinical course of acute infections was described in detail.

In the preface the authors set out that the publisher had informed them that a concise, practical work on dealing with sick children was a desideratum in the British medical literature. Evanson wrote chapters on the peculiarities of the infant structure and constitution, the general considerations involved, digestive organs, organs of respiration, circulation, cerebral spinal system, locomotor apparatus and growth. Maunsell wrote chapters on management immediately after birth, food and medicine, food in the first period, choice of a nurse, artificial feeding, weaning, food in the second period, cleanliness, clothing, sleep, exercise, medicine, light, air, temperature, and mental and moral education.

Reviews in other medical journals were also enthusiastic. An anonymous *Dublin Journal of Medical Science* reviewer said that the medical profession was indebted to the authors. Maunsell was Professor of Obstetrics in Dublin

University but in 1841 he became Professor of Hygiene and Political Medicine and established a reputation as a pioneering advocate of what came to be known as social medicine.[31] Evanson became Professor of Medicine in the Royal College of Surgeons in 1836.

OUTPATIENT AND INPATIENT SERVICES

At first all the patients were treated on an outpatient basis. In 1834 there were no beds in service. In that year Evanson reported a case of suspected inhalation of a fishbone. The child was brought to the Institution but the parents were told to bring the child to the Meath Hospital as 'at the Institution for Children accommodation for intern patients is not provided'.[32] There was a similar lack of accommodation recorded in 1843.[33] Dominic Corrigan, giving evidence to a Select Committee of the House of Commons, gave a list of eighteen Dublin hospitals described as medical charities; and the list does not include the Institution for the Diseases of Children, according to Hansard.[34] The extern services had, however, acquired an international reputation and in this capacity the Institution flourished, with annual patient attendances of 7,000 or more.

In 1850 the *Dublin Pictorial Guide and Directory* listed the address as 8 and 9 Pitt Street, occupying two houses rather than one. In 1852 the *Medical Directory* entry also recorded a change of name. The Institution was now described as the Hospital for the Diseases of Children and for the first time a matron was named, a Mrs Bagnall. The entries in the *Medical Directory* continued to use the designation 'Hospital' to describe it each year until 1864. The increase in the floor area, now utilizing the accommodation of two extensive houses, and the appointment of a matron, both suggest that inpatients were now catered for. *The Dublin Hospital Gazette* for 1859 also describes the Institution as a hospital. Unfortunately the census records for 1851 and 1861 have been destroyed and cannot be consulted to confirm the social profile of the contemporary inpatients. A similar problem emerges from a review of the contemporary Dublin and London medical journals. The review has not brought to light any case report that could definitively confirm that a particular patient was an inpatient in the Institution.

In 1863 the *Medical Directory* reverted to the use of the term Institution. These changes probably indicate that inpatients were expected to be admitted from 1852 to 1863 and that intended or existing inpatient services were then phased out again. They were regenerated in 1886 when the Institution merged with the National Orthopaedic Hospital to form the forty-bed National Children's Hospital, on the site in Harcourt Street where it continued in an expanded form until its relocation to the Tallaght Hospital site in 1998.

RELATIONSHIP BETWEEN THE CHILDREN'S HOSPITAL AND THE MEATH HOSPITAL

To a degree the Meath Hospital and the Hospital for Children were complementary. In 1864 the Smyly Ward, a designated children's ward, was opened in the Meath Hospital.[35] William Stokes (1804–77) was at that time consulting physician both to the Hospital for the Diseases of Children and to the Meath Hospital, in which he was the lead clinician and was responsible for the medical instruction of students. A man of great distinction, he was a Fellow of the King's and Queen's College of Physicians, Regius Professor of the Theory and Practice of Medicine in Dublin University and Examiner in the Practice of Medicine in the Queen's University of Ireland. Also serving as visiting physicians were Samuel Hardy (1815-1868), an obstetrician, and John William Moore (1845–1937). In 1875 Moore succeeded William Stokes as lead clinician in the Meath Hospital. A former pupil of Stokes', he re-edited Stokes' textbook on fevers in 1876. He went on to make a major contribution to paediatric hospital care in Dublin.

STOKES' OPINION OF CHILDREN'S HOSPITALS

Stokes' role in limiting the function of the Children's Hospital can be inferred from his speech at the opening of the Smyly Ward for children in the Meath Hospital in 1864.[36] He clearly had divided loyalties. He said: 'Without impugning the value of children's hospitals it might be asked whether special hospitals for the diseases of children are to be preferred to the allocation of wards for similar problems in a great general hospital.' Referring to the choice between a children's hospital and a children's ward in a general hospital he said that this was one of those questions that must be 'solved by experience'. He went on to say:

> In the meantime I may be permitted to express my opinion that of the two plans the latter is the preferable one. The powers of the human mind become narrowed whenever they are long confined to any one specialty. Great physicians and great surgeons are only made by practice in a general hospital. In a hospital exclusively devoted to infantile diseases it is not likely that its inmates could ever have the advantage of such judgment and skill as that possessed by a Cooper, a Baillie, a Crampton or a Cheyne ... The establishment of a children's ward or wards is a matter greatly to be desired in every large hospital.

Stokes was clearly of the opinion that the inpatient service hitherto provided by the Children's Hospital could be improved upon by now providing it in the new children's ward at the Meath Hospital. He nevertheless remained listed in the *Medical Directory* as consulting physician to the Institution on a continuing basis from 1864 until he retired in 1874.

CHILDREN'S HOSPITAL CHAMPION

Stokes was challenged at the Smyly Ward opening by the Lord Lieutenant in Ireland, Lord John Wodehouse (1826–1902). Wodehouse stated that those who devoted themselves to special departments acquired particular knowledge that was not possessed by others who travelled over a wider field. He said:

> I believe that where you have these special hospitals on a large scale you advance medical science more effectually than through having professional duties extended over too wide a field. I think that all who have attended to the progress we have

made in the various sciences must perceive that those who have dedicated themselves to some special pursuit are generally those who have made new discoveries and inventions for the benefit of mankind.

Lord Wodehouse had previously held a post in the diplomatic corps at the court of the Tsar in St Petersburg and so he was familiar with the St Petersburg Children's Hospital which had been founded in 1834. Members of the Wodehouse family are on the list of subscribers to Great Ormond Street Children's Hospital in London.

PHYSICIANS AS PAEDIATRICIANS

Because of worries about cross-infection, many authorities recommended that young children should be mixed with adult patients and special wards for children should be avoided. For this reason it was the custom to admit young children to women's wards and boys over the age of seven to men's wards.[37] In consequence the children in the general hospitals came under the care of the distinguished physicians of the day. Stokes himself reported on his experience of convulsions in 1832 before there was a children's ward in the Meath Hospital and, indeed, before he was appointed to the Institution for Diseases of Children.[38] Dominic Corrigan (1802–80) wrote extensively on pica in children from Jervis Street Hospital in 1859.[39] However, he also advocated a rather bizarre method of treating enuretic boys by sealing the urethra at night with collodion.[40] John Crampton (1768–1840), King's Professor of Materia Medica and physician to Dr Steevens' Hospital and the Hardwicke Hospital, has already been referred to as one of the founding fathers of the Institution.

In 1875 John William Moore succeeded William Stokes in the Meath Hospital and he contributed greatly to the treatment of children there. He did not, however, take on Stokes' commitment to the Institution. In the Meath Hospital he continued to make a major contribution to the understanding of childhood illness.

CHILDREN'S WARDS IN DUBLIN HOSPITALS (SEE APPENDIX AT END OF CHAPTER)

In spite of the forebodings about infection, a children's ward was opened in St Vincent's Hospital in Dublin in 1836, described in the *Medical Directory* as being based on the Hospice des Enfants Malades in Paris, which had been founded in 1802. A major effort was made to interest the St Vincent's medical students in childhood illness. Each year the *Medical Directory*'s hospital entry advertised a special prize offered by Dr O'Ferral for the best paper presented by a student on a series of paediatric cases. The City of Dublin Hospital opened a children's ward in 1838. This maintained its clinical momentum up to the end of the nineteenth century, when Langford Symes, a member of staff, dominated the clinical arena in Dublin. In his publications he is described as pathologist and assistant physician to the hospital, but he is not listed in the definitive history of the institution.[41] His interests were clinical and he published fifteen papers on paediatric subjects. He had trained in Great Ormond Street, and he was probably the first Dublin paediatrician. He conducted a national survey of infant mortality, comparing the figures for the major towns.[42]

Symes became the attending physician to the children of the viceroy, Lord Dudley, during the years 1902–5. His numerous contributions to the paediatric literature dominated the *Dublin Journal of Medical Science* during the first twenty years of the twentieth century.

As well as the Smyly Ward in the Meath Hospital, children's wards were opened in the Adelaide Hospital in 1881 and in Sir Patrick Dun's Hospital in 1882. St Joseph's Infirmary, a freestanding independent children's hospital, first opened its doors in Buckingham Street in 1872. When the Irish Sisters of Charity took it over in 1876 the children's ward in St Vincent's Hospital, also run by the Sisters, was no longer heavily promoted.

THE MEATH HOSPITAL CONNECTION WITH THE INSTITUTION FOR DISEASES OF CHILDREN

Stokes himself maintained an interest in the children admitted to the Smyly Ward over the years, but in 1885 the Smyly Ward became designated as a surgical ward and there was no children's ward in the hospital until a new one was built in 1877. This was the year in which the Institution for Diseases of Children merged with the Orthopaedic Hospital, leading ultimately to the establishment of a forty-bed paediatric hospital in Harcourt Street. The knowledge that the Institution now included a large inpatient facility presumably triggered a decision to ensure that the Meath Hospital was able to provide similar facilities.

Children had, however, always been admitted to the fever wards and to adult medical wards. This continued under Sir John William Moore, who had succeeded Stokes in 1875. Moore belonged to the fourth generation of a medical dynasty, and indeed the medical tradition would continue in the family through yet another five generations.[43] By coincidence Moore's father William D. Moore, an apothecary turned physician, was listed as physician to the Institution for Disease of Children from 1864 until his death in 1871. In 1926, at the age of 78, John Moore gave an introductory address at the opening of the teaching programme in the Meath Hospital in which he spoke on the treatment of children.[44] He was still clinically active, but in the absence of a children's medical ward 74 of the 114 children reported on were on the fever wing and 70 children were treated on adult medical wards of the Meath Hospital.[45]

Moore advocated breastfeeding and home hygiene and he decried the fact that the Leinster Lawn was no longer open as a children's playground for the children of the inner city. Speaking later of sick children he also said: 'A doctor, if he is to succeed in the treatment of children, has to be able to capture the fortress of a child's heart. He should have a smile on his lips, or better still, in his eyes, and his watchword should be "faith, hope and love, the greatest of which was love"'. He was an advocate of the notification of infectious disease and of the isolation of infectious cases. Speaking of doctors' responsibility he said:

> No other calling, the church not excepted, demands so much
> self-denial, patience, and with reverence I say it, prayer. Armed

with such a panoply, the physician is fully equipped for the battle with disease and death ... Should he suffer defeat in what may prove to be an unequal conflict, vanquished he may indeed be, but with untarnished armour and without disgrace. And yet are not all of us in a very special sense still medical students? Not a day passes in our professional life that an opportunity does not offer of learning something new, of testing that something and making use thereof.

He had wide-ranging interests and two years later he wrote an analysis of epidemiology in Ireland.[46] He was knighted by Queen Victoria in 1911 for his services to medicine. During his lifetime he published more than 150 medical papers.

GEORGE FLEETWOOD CHURCHILL

In 1869 the *Medical Directory* listed Dr George Fleetwood Churchill as physician to the Institution. He graduated from the Royal College of Surgeons in 1862 and he was elected a Fellow of the College of Physicians of Ireland in 1868. He was also physician to the Clergy Daughters' School and later was appointed to the visiting staff of the Magdalene Asylum, Miss Carr's Homes and other charities. He had the good fortune to be the son of Fleetwood Churchill, Professor of Midwifery in the King's and Queen's Royal College of Physicians and President of the Dublin Obstetric Society.

Professor Fleetwood Churchill was best known for his textbook on the diseases of women, but in 1858, having diligently scoured the world literature, he produced another textbook entitled the *Diseases of Children*.[47] He himself had not had direct contact with sick children and the book was criticized. *The Lancet* reviewer wrote that if the directions in the book were followed, a great deal of mischief would be done.[48] The book, however, sold well in the United States and Fleetwood Churchill was made an honorary member of the American National Institute and of the Philadelphia Medical Society. A second edition was published under his own name but for the third and final edition published in 1970, his son George Fleetwood Churchill emerged as co-author. His father retired in 1874 and George did not produce any further edition of the book. George continued as a member of the staff of the Institution until his death. Dying in 1884, he did not live to see the Institution move to its new site.

THE DUBLIN INFLUENCE IN ENGLAND

Although William Stokes was on the staff of the Children's Hospital, he never recorded this in his personal entries in the *Medical Directory* and he undoubtedly regarded this appointment as being subsidiary to his appointment to the Meath Hospital. He was probably unaware of the extent to which the Dublin Institution had directly influenced developments in England. Charles West, the founder of Great Ormond Street Hospital in London, attended the Rotunda Hospital in 1838 and, according to his obituary, he divided his time between obstetrics and paediatrics. More than ten years after his Rotunda visit, his interest in Dublin medicine was maintained and he bought the 1847 second edition of the textbook of paediatrics published from the Institution by Maunsell and Evanson.[49] They had both been in post when he visited Dublin. The text is among the surviving volumes of his personal library still held in Great Ormond Street Hospital. Ten other Dublin books are in the collection. In his *Lectures on the Diseases of Childhood* he referred in several places to the clinical views of Stokes, Graves and Crampton.[50] He also referred with enthusiasm to Kennedy's 1843 account of his experience of the treatment of scarlet fever.[51]

The foundation of the Liverpool Children's Infirmary has also been ascribed to the visit to Dublin in 1843 of Alfred Stephens, the founding father of the Infirmary.[52] Birmingham was another city that benefited from a Dublin contact. Thomas Pretious Heslop, the founder of Birmingham Children's Hospital, had been a clinical clerk in the Meath Hospital for a year and he spoke very highly of the training he received there from Stokes, although he does not specifically refer to the Institution for the Diseases of Children.[53] In effect this appears to confirm Stokes' perception that his work in the children's ward of his main hospital took precedence over his connection with the Institution for Diseases of Children.

With the passage of time the National Children's Hospital in Harcourt Street consolidated its position as a reputable centre of excellence in the paediatric field, with universally respected clinical staff.[54] Professor Robert Steen, appointed to the new University of Dublin Chair of Paediatrics in 1960, was President of the British Paediatric Association in 1968. In 1973, at a meeting of the Association of the Professors of Paediatrics in Keswick, at which the Trinity College Dublin and University College Dublin chair holders attended, the eminent Professor Ronald Illingworth made the suggestion that the paediatric departments of University College Dublin and Dublin University together with their associated children's hospitals should merge on one site. He had been the external assessor for the two recent paediatric academic appointments in each of the universities and he had conducted two evaluations of Dublin paediatrics. After prolonged discussion the concept of a merger was ultimately agreed by all concerned, but this was blocked by Archbishop Dermot Ryan, the nominator of the management committee of Our Lady's Hospital for Sick Children (f. 1956). The failure of the amalgamation ultimately led to the relocation of the National Children's Hospital to Tallaght to join the Meath and the Adelaide Hospitals on a new site. At the present time (2012), the integration of the children's hospitals is again under consideration.

APPENDIX
CHRONOLOGY OF CHILDREN'S CLINICS, WARDS AND HOSPITALS IN DUBLIN

1822	Outpatient clinics, Dublin Institution for the Diseases of Children, No. 9 Pitt Street
1832	Children's Ward, St Vincent's Hospital
1850–63	Outpatients/Inpatients Dublin Hospital for the Diseases of Children, Nos 8–9 Pitt Street (formerly the Institution for the Diseases of Children)
1858	Children's Ward, City of Dublin Hospital
1864	Dublin Hospital, the Diseases of Children re-designated as the Institution for the Diseases of Children
1864	Smyly Children's Ward, Meath Hospital, re-designated as a surgical ward in 1885 and a new children's ward was built
1872	Opening of St Joseph's infirmary in Buckingham Street
1879	St Joseph's Infirmary moved to Temple Street, renamed Children's Hospital
1881	Children's Ward, Adelaide Hospital
1886	Merger of Institution for Diseases of Children and National Orthopaedic Hospital, renamed National Children's Hospital
1887	Children's Ward, Dr Steevens' Hospital

3

The Gentle Application of Mercury: Treatment of Children at the Westmoreland Lock Hospital, Dublin, in the Mid-Nineteenth Century

Jean M. Walker

*B*abies and children with congenital or acquired syphilis are among the least visible of all of the syphilitic patients who attended the Westmoreland Lock Hospital (WLH), Dublin.[1] The WLH was a hospital established under charter for the treatment of sexually transmitted disease among the indigent and pauper population of Dublin, forming part of the city's medical network from 1792 to 1955. Publicity of all kinds was eschewed by its governors in order to protect the privacy of patients due to the nature of the diseases treated, and its patients were regarded with varying degrees of moral outrage and sympathy during the course of the nineteenth century. This chapter brings into focus the treatment of children (from infancy to 15 years of age) at the WLH through exploration of a number of key issues. The undoubted presence of children at the WLH was rarely overtly acknowledged in the nineteenth century, and this chapter explores why this was the case. The extent to which doctors perceived their role as one of guardianship over their young patients, taking personal responsibility for the recovery of these patients, will be considered. The chapter also asks whether the level of medical care expended on children was influenced by the poor prognosis, short life expectancy and visible signs of morbidity displayed by them.

The question of whether children in particular were exploited in the institution on account of their precarious social position will be discussed in respect of their involvement in trials of treatment and experimental research. These trials were carried out in the WLH during the tenure of Dr John Morgan (1868–76), whose series of experimental inoculations included as subjects a number of very young girls.[2] The case histories and observations Morgan presented of his WLH patients are central sources referred to in order to demonstrate how doctors perceived poor syphilitic children throughout the period in question.

SOURCES OF INFORMATION ABOUT CHILDREN IN THE WLH

The archives of the WLH are held by the Royal College of Physicians of Ireland (RCPI) in Kildare Street, Dublin and reveal incidental details that illuminate brief periods of the lives of those mentioned within them.[3] However, very little of this information relates to children who resided in the hospital, either as patients or newborns, with limited details concerning children's medical treatment or accommodation. Information regarding infants born in the hospital, who were brought there by their mothers or who died in there, is contained within the 'observations' column of the general register of admissions. This column was used to record incidental information concerning the patient but was not utilized as a matter of course. The frequency of observations most likely depended on the diligence of the registrar at the time and the information available to him. The 'observations' column is particularly detailed for the years 1864 and 1865, and data from these years forms the basis of this chapter. Admission registers for the WLH are not extant after 1868.[4]

This lack of detail makes it necessary to look at published medical literature for information regarding attitudes to syphilitic children at the WLH. A number of WLH doctors contributed to expert discussion within medical journals and texts throughout the nineteenth century. Many doctors who became venereal specialists in Ireland underwent some of their training in this hospital, which only intermittently admitted medical students during the nineteenth century. In the early years of its existence, the distinguished surgeon Abraham Colles worked at the hospital. He was president of the Royal College of Surgeons in Ireland (RCSI) in 1802 and in this capacity was on the WLH's board of governors in that year. His observations of mothers and babies at the hospital were the basis on which he formed his famous medical 'laws' about the contagious nature of syphilis. These laws were published in 1837 and stated that a child with syphilis would infect its wet nurse but not its own mother.[5] Philip Crampton, who became a major figure in the development of public health in Ireland, similarly drew upon his experiences in the WLH in his work.[6] Richard Carmichael (1776–1849) was assistant surgeon to the WLH in 1810 and a governor in 1813 when president of the RCSI. In this year he gave a series of lectures to medical students at the WLH. He wrote a number of monographs on syphilis and was considered eminent in this field by the ground-breaking French venereologist Anton Ricord.[7] Thomas Byrne, surgeon at the WLH (1833–69), studied in Ricord's hospital in Paris in the 1830s. Ricord's theories were quoted in all the general works on syphilis and debates on the control of sexually transmitted diseases in Great Britain into the 1870s. Paul Diday, a French doctor who was one of the first to make a particular study of infantile syphilis, referred to the work of Irish doctors John Cruise Egan, James William Cusack and Abraham Colles.[8] All of these doctors used case histories of WLH patients in their discussions of syphilis and its treatment. WLH doctors and governors also gave evidence to committees of enquiry on venereal diseases,[9] particularly the series relating to the introduction and operation of the Contagious Diseases Acts ((CDA) 1864, 1866 and 1869 – repealed in 1886). These acts were intended to arrest the spread of sexually transmitted disease among army and navy personnel by subjecting women in up to eighteen specified naval ports and army garrison towns in Britain and Ireland to compulsory fortnightly internal examination if they were suspected of being prostitutes and to periods of up to three months in a 'lock' ward if they were found to be diseased.[10] As Ireland was part of the 'home station', bases were controlled by the British War Office, and Ireland was included in this legislation. Irish military, religious and medical men gave evidence at each enquiry. In England, fifteen areas were subject to the CDA and in Ireland, the Curragh, Cork and Cobh were classified areas. Some of the evidence given by witnesses called before the first committee of enquiry suggested that as syphilis was passed on to a sufferer's children, 'a serious national consideration is involved in the subject'[11] and was responsible for the degeneration of the children of the nation ultimately posing a threat to the future security of Great Britain by 'spreading wide its evil consequences over the population, and especially over the seaports and garrison towns'.[12] Later enquiries debated the possibility of extending the jurisdiction of the acts to more naval and military bases and to some civilian areas with large numbers of prostitutes, especially London and Dublin.[13] WLH doctors and governors had a particular interest in this question and many favoured the extension of the Contagious Diseases Acts to Dublin. Others were insistent that the voluntary admission and discharge policy of the WLH was intrinsic to its ethos, but were nevertheless in favour of compelling patients to complete their treatment within the hospital once they had been admitted.

THE SYPHILITIC CONDITION AND TREATMENT OF CHILDREN AT THE WLH

Three categories of sick children were treated at the WLH: those who were born to women who were already patients in the hospital, coming under treatment after their birth; those who were born ostensibly healthy but who later developed signs of syphilitic infection;[14] and those with acquired syphilis, possibly infected through wet-nursing, or through petting or kissing an infected infant or an older care-giver. The only other children admitted were infants at the breast, who, in the absence of wet-nursing or artificial feeding facilities, could not be left in the care of anyone but their mother.

Infants with syphilis often looked very different from healthy babies. In the mid-nineteenth century, Diday likened a syphilitic infant to 'nothing more than a little wrinkled old man with a cold in his head'.[15] The description was of such accuracy and had such resonance for doctors that it has not been surpassed and is still quoted in modern medical textbooks.[16] The peculiar snuffly breathing of the babies was due to the fact that the nasal cartilage was foreshortened, making breathing difficult. The teeth, when they grew, were short and square and had distinctive excoriations. These teeth were one of the signs of later congenital syphilis and, together with interstitial keratitis and nerve deafness, have since been called 'Hutchinson's triad'.[17] Often affected babies were stillborn or died at or soon after birth; were weak and puny with little ability to suck and a consequent failure to thrive; and had a distinctive shrill cry that was apparently unmistakable. Babies affected before birth and born exhibiting signs of florid syphilis had a particular smell, which was most unpleasant and has been described by modern medical practitioners as 'quite unforgettable'.[18] Sometimes babies were asymptomatic at birth, but developed signs of syphilis within a short number of weeks. The first sign of disease in an infant was often lesions at mouth and anus, while later they might be observed to suffer hearing and mental impairment.[19] Morgan noted that 'eruption appears as a murkiness about the mouth, face and chin; the general colour is earthy, and the face aged-looking'.[20] None of these descriptions, however, are as evocative as the description of an untreated child when 'the child is reduced to a state of excessive debility, and dies, covered with disgusting scabs and ulcerations'.[21] The possibility of relief from such a disease was likely to have provided a strong incentive to bring a child to the WLH. Between the WLH's establishment in 1792 and 1820, men, women and children were admitted to the hospital. In 1817, the first full year for which a hospital admissions register exists, more women were admitted than men, and less than 10 per cent of these women were accompanied by children (see Table 1).

Table 1. Number and Percentages of Admissions and Deaths of Patients in the Westmoreland Lock Hospital, 1 January to 31 December 1817 and 1 January to 31 December 1819

Year	Number and % of total admissions				Number and % of total deaths			
	1817		1819		1817		1819	
	No.	%	No	%	No	%	No	%
Women	794	50	861	52.4	7	41.1	11	61.1
Men	728	45.8	743	45.2	8	47.1	4	22.2
Child and mother	54	3.4	33	2	2	11.8	3	16.7
Child with man	9	0.5	1	0.6	0		0	0
Child alone	2	0.1	4	0.24	0		0	0
Total	1587		1642		17		18	

Source: General Register of Patients 1817-27, WLH Archive, RCPI, Dublin.

In 1817 nine children came to the hospital with their father. Only two children were unaccompanied by any adult. No details were recorded of their illness, their age or their address, but they were most likely sent to the WLH from orphanages or poorhouses in the city. A father might have brought his child to the WLH because the mother was dead, she was not ill enough to be admitted, she was caring for other children or she was in another institution. Two years later, in 1819 (the next year for which substantial admissions are recorded), the trend remained largely the same. Although the total admissions were higher, only one child was accompanied by a male.

The only comparable institution in the early nineteenth century, St John's Fever and Lock Hospital, Limerick, had a system of sponsorship recording occupation and address as well as details of illness.[22] However, because the WLH noted only name, age and date of admission, it is necessary to extrapolate: if a 3-year-old entered the hospital unaccompanied or with its father, then it must have been diseased; if a 10-month-old attended with its mother, it may or may not have been the subject of treatment.

Between 1819 and 1955 when the hospital closed, there was very restricted entry for children and only adult females were admitted. During this period, boys up to the age of 5 were accepted into the hospital only when accompanied by their mother. Those not eligible for admission to the WLH were accommodated in Sir Patrick Dun's Hospital, Dr Steevens' Hospital and the Richmond Hospital.

In the earliest days of its foundation, a male *accoucheur* was retained by the WLH, but in later years, if a labour was uncomplicated, the child was delivered by nurses who claimed a fee for midwifery duties. In cases where complications arose, the resident surgeon or midwife would attend the patient. By 1900, the midwifery nurse was required to have certification, and was one of the few nursing staff who was trained. Where possible, when a woman presented at the WLH in labour she was sent immediately to a maternity hospital where they were obliged to accept any woman in labour even if she were syphilitic or a prostitute. In Dublin, the Coombe Lying-In Hospital (established 1829) and the Rotunda Hospital (established 1745) catered without censure for poor pregnant women.[23] Both received cases of syphilitic women attending for the births of their babies. It was claimed at the Poor Inquiry Commission of 1834 that the high number of stillbirths at the Coombe Hospital was due to the prevalence of venereal disease among the poorest families of the city.[24] Often a mother and her infant would be sent to the WLH post-delivery, where they would be treated for syphilis. In this way the WLH limited the number of maternity cases to those where the mother had been under treatment before the birth (see Table 2).

Given that in the general population a large proportion of pregnancies in syphilitic mothers ended in miscarriage or stillbirth, the number of mothers with surviving children presenting at the WLH for treatment would always be far lower than the number of women who had previously borne children who were admitted. The registrar-general for Ireland, Sir William Thompson, demonstrated that 912 children under the age of 1 in Ireland whose deaths were certified in the twenty-year period 1881–1900 were assigned congenital syphilis as a cause of death. He showed that this equated to 8.5 per cent of registered births in this period. Due to a number of factors such as a general

Table 2. Infants born in the Westmoreland Lock Hospital, 1877-83

Year	Syphilitic Infants born alive		Syphilitic Infants stillborn		Total syphilitic births
1877-8	5	41.6%	7	58.3%	12
1878-9	8	66.6%	4	33.3%	12
1879-80	7	63.6%	4	36.3%	11
1880-1	13	54.1%	11	45.8%	24
1881-2	11	47.8%	12	52.1%	23
1882-3	11	47.8%	12	52.1%	23
Total	55	47.6%	50	52.4%	105

Source: *Board of Superintendence of Dublin Hospitals 25th Annual Report, Appendix 1*, p. 23.

under-registration of infant births and deaths in the earlier part of this period, and the reluctance of doctors to register syphilis as a cause of death, it is likely that the actual number of infant deaths from congenital syphilis was considerably higher than Thompson's estimate.[25] Neither syphilitic babies brought to hospital for treatment nor babies born with congenital syphilis and under treatment were recorded as patients in the WLH's statistics until 1885 and they were thus not included in the mortality statistics compiled for the Board of Superintendence prior to this date.

As demonstrated in Table 3, between 1885 and 1900 there were 218 births and 216 deaths in the hospital. It is unclear whether these death statistics included stillbirths.

Frequently a mother left the WLH soon after her child's death, suggesting that she had only remained there so that the child would get proper treatment and warmth. In these cases, it is unlikely that the mother herself was under treatment. For instance, Catherine Waters came to the hospital with her 4-day-old diseased baby and when he died she left 'to bury her child'.[26] Similarly, Mary Conroy attended the hospital for six days and left on the day her child died, while Catherine Hayes stayed in the hospital for three days and was discharged on the day her 5-month-old

Table 3. Figures for Admissions, Deaths and Births at the Westmoreland Lock Hospital, 1885-1900

Year	Admissions	Deaths		Births	
1885	754	25	3.32%	22	2.92%
1886	739	15	2.03%	12	1.62%
1887	661	13	1.97%	13	1.97%
1888	624	13	2.08%	17	2.72%
1889	594	14	2.36%	15	2.53%
1890	630	14	2.22%	16	2.54%
1891	635	10	1.57%	15	2.36%
1892	577	18	3.12%	9	1.56%
1893	646	17	2.63%	12	1.86%
1894	635	15	2.36%	12	1.89%
1895	490	11	2.24%	17	3.47%
1896	416	5	1.20%	11	2.64%
1897	386	14	3.63%	14	3.63%
1898	427	10	2.34%	9	2.11%
1899	417	14	3.36%	11	2.64%
1900	473	8	1.69%	13	2.75%
Total	9104	216		218	

Source: *Board of Superintendence of Dublin Hospitals, 28th to 42nd Annual Reports.*

child died.[27] Data submitted to the Board of Superintendence over the period 1886–92 provides evidence that this was a longstanding practice. The classification in the annual return of hospital admissions of 'undiseased mothers with diseased children and diseased mothers with undiseased children' suggests that if the diseased child died, the mother, who was only in the hospital to care for her child, would be required to leave immediately (see Table 4). This cumbersome classification was dispensed with after 1892. Some female children were admitted during 1864 and 1865 unaccompanied by their mothers. In these cases, the girls were suffering from gonorrhoea. Rosanna Courtney was aged 10 when she attended the WLH

Table 4 Undiseased and Diseased Mothers and Infants admitted to the Westmoreland Lock Hospital, 1886-92

	1886	1887	1888	1889	1890	1891	1892
Undiseased mothers admitted with diseased children	10					6	7
Undiseased infants admitted with diseased mothers	11					15	4
Both categories of infants and mothers		7	17	25	28		
Undiseased infants born in hospital							9
Total	21	7	17	25	28	21	20

Source: *Board of Superintendence of Dublin Hospitals 28th-34th Annual Reports.*

and was discharged 'cured' into the care of her mother.[28] She is the youngest female listed in 1864 or 1865. Twelve-year-old Ellen MacAuley also attended the hospital unaccompanied and was discharged into the care of her mother.[29]

Although it appears that babies were given considerable care and attention in order to cure or relieve their symptoms, comments about children are sparse in the hospital registers. For example, in the annual accounts there is no mention of the provision of nursery accommodation, or of the purchase of cots or cradles or any other paraphernalia, nor are there any details provided about particular medical preparations given to babies. There is no comment made about conditions for children or infants in the forty-three years of inspections at the hospital from 1857 to 1900, although a child dietary was included in the returns of diet as part of the Board of Superintendence inspections. This consisted of one pint of 'new milk' and six ounces of bread per day given out at breakfast, with 'new milk' or one ounce of arrowroot or sago with sugar or beef tea, given out as an extra at dinner time if they were prescribed. The dietary does not appear to have been altered until the twentieth century. This silence regarding a considerable cohort of the hospital population points to their insignificance as far as the managerial and medical authorities of the hospital were concerned.

MEDICAL TREATMENT AND EXPERIMENTAL TRIALS ON CHILDREN

Babies with congenital syphilis could be treated with potassium iodide, chlorate of potash, or creosote.[30] They were also often treated with mercury in either oral or topical forms. Mercury was seen as the most effective solution for syphilis – even for babies – in spite of the considerable side effects. Children were often given far smaller doses than adults, for shorter periods.[31] Sometimes the colour and smell of mercurial treatments would be disguised to make them more tolerable to children.[32] Often they were wrapped in a silk tube saturated with a mercurial compound. This treatment originated with Benjamin Brodie in the London Lock Hospital. This silk tube, known as 'Brodie's stocking', was slipped over the leg or body of the infant and left in place until the mercury took effect. Thomas Byrne said: 'I treat them with what is called "Brodie's stocking", feeding them well at the same time, and you see the disease retiring under your very eye.'[33] Newborn infants' eyes were routinely dropped with silver nitrate to offset the blinding disease iritis, which was a severe danger to children born of mothers who had active syphilis with lesions in the birth canal. Morgan commented: 'In the insidious iritis of infants, the gentle use of mercury either by inunction or its internal administration must be had recourse to without delay.'[34] In spite of Morgan's phraseology, it must be noted that the effects of mercury on the infant would have been in no way 'gentle'.[35]

Babies were treated with humanity and compassion when doctors were alert to family circumstance. Byrne was in the habit of recording the life story of every person admitted to the WLH.[36] He declared:

> On a late occasion I showed to a gentleman, who is an advocate
> for a different mode of treating infantile venereal disease,

three babies of about two months or ten weeks old. They were apparently in rude health, and finer children could not be seen. I told him that these children six weeks before were labouring under venereal disease, and they were then apparently cured. He said that it was only apparently so, and that in a few years they would be attacked with bad forms of disease. I entered my protest against that assertion, because I have seen some of these babies, when grown up, come to our hospital years afterwards with their mothers, being then strong, healthy children.[37]

The visiting doctor's comment to Byrne is indicative of his view that affected children would never remain well. This statement also reveals that WLH doctors were not working in isolation, but were discussing all forms of treatment of congenital syphilis with their professional colleagues. They observed the health of the babies in their care and were anxious to demonstrate their success in curing a condition where affected children could undergo various treatments until they eventually died of emaciation and exhaustion.[38] Byrne ultimately expressed his opinion of the WLH when he left a number of bequests in his will, including one to the Protestant Orphan Asylum. Yet he did not leave a bequest to the institution where he worked for almost forty years.[39]

TRIALS OF INOCULATION IN THE WLH

It was during Byrne's tenure that Morgan was appointed to the hospital. He was interested in the origin of sexually transmitted diseases, speculating as to whether they were all caused by the same 'germ' and attempting to discern the usefulness of inoculation against syphilis. The cause and treatment of syphilis remained a vexed question until the discoveries of the *Treponema pallidum* spirochaetes by Shaudinn and Hoffman in 1905 and of Salvarsan by Paul Ehrlich in 1905.[40]

In 1870 two 8-year-old girls were admitted to the WLH. Morgan considered them such suitable candidates for his experiments that he brought them to the

Obstetrical Society of Ireland to illustrate his work. In the first case, he said the girl was 'suffering only from vulval condylomata, with a very clean and clear skin'.[41] He inoculated her on the abdomen with the vaginal secretion of another patient. After a month, Morgan said: 'There is still a general murkiness of skin … The second inoculated sore shows as yet but little inclination to heal.'[42] The second child was also inoculated with the vaginal secretion of another patient. The resulting sore was observed and drawn. Morgan used matter from this sore to inoculate other subjects. His final observation was succinct, that 'the health of the girl rapidly improved, and the condylomata healed, but the artificial chancroid still exists'.[43] Morgan's case history noted that the child was infected by her sister, who was married to a man with 'mucous patches' on his mouth. He contracted the infection through illicit sexual activity and introduced it to his family in the course of normal conjugal activity with his wife. The child was subsequently infected by his wife. The wife and her young sister were both victims in this case, while the child was further objectified by her use as a scientific subject at the hands of the medical profession.

There is no suggestion that Morgan obtained permission from parents or guardians of any young patients prior to the use of experimental treatments. However, the ethical idea of seeking parental permission or informed consent before subjecting a child to questionable treatments and display before a medical audience would not necessarily have occurred to the surgeon, given the hospital rules' stipulation that patients who objected to treatments would be summarily discharged. Morgan could also have been influenced by the CDA discourse, which gave doctors complete control over women who were brought to government lock hospitals.[44]

Morgan was ordered to desist from his experimental treatments by the governors at the WLH, who resolved that 'the inoculation of the patients with the virus of the venereal disease be discontinued in this hospital'.[45] They added that if Morgan wished to continue such experiments he must get official sanction from the lord lieutenant, who declined to get involved as he considered it to be a medical matter in which Morgan should adhere to the wishes of the hospital governors.[46] Morgan was considerably annoyed by this decision, which he considered a greatly missed opportunity, both for himself and for medical science generally.[47] He argued passionately that his treatment was justified by the greater good, and compared his work to that being carried out by Professor Carl Wilhelm Boeck at the University of Christiana in Norway and Professor Freeman J. Bumstead in America.[48] He pointed out how little was known about how smallpox inoculation worked in the human system and yet it had already brought huge changes to public health. Morgan considered the potential effect of his work to be of similar importance. He stressed that the inoculation itself caused little discomfort, being made only with the point of a pin, and that he experimented only on patients who were already contaminated by venereal disease, so that there was no risk of the 'syphilitic poison' being accidentally disseminated into a healthy person. This argument for the legitimacy of using infected patients in trials of treatment was not unusual at the time.[49] The negative response by the WLH governors to his work demonstrates their fear that Morgan's work would bring unwelcome publicity to the hospital and that women, who came voluntarily to the hospital, would resist admission if they felt they would be subjected to experimental treatment. This would counteract the governors' objective in preventing the spread of syphilis by diseased females who might otherwise be treated at the WLH.

THE STIGMATIZATION OF SYPHILIS AND PATIENTS OF THE WLH

In 1872 Morgan published a textbook on syphilis with case histories and illustrations of patients from the WLH and other hospitals in which he also considered a number of what he called 'medico-legal' questions. On the question of whether the disease could pass from diseased father to foetus without infecting the mother, he came to the conclusion that in some cases this was possible, but that the reverse could also occur.[50] Culpability of the parents for the infection of wet nurses by an infected nursling was also discussed. Such cases often involved private middle-class families in disputes that brought issues of sexual transgression, infection of spouses and the 'hereditary' notion of syphilis into the public domain.[51] This also indicates how privately treated middle-class women could be kept in ignorance of their condition through collusion between their husband and doctor.[52] Morgan also 'deplored' what he called 'amateur wet-nursing' or the 'interchange of babies', which he claimed took place in crowded households.[53]

Morgan explained how he came to treat a 68-year-old woman who was outside the normal age range of his patients: 'a married, respectable woman, became infected by patches from the grandchild's mouth ... The father of the child, "a hard-working mechanic", had been affected by primary [syphilis] five years before, and the mother had constitutional signs only'.[54] In this scenario, the infected man marrying into the family had contaminated his wife, her mother and his child.[55] The grandmother, mother and child all became patients of the hospital, suggesting that this was a lower- rather than middle-class family. This case history had already been referred to by Morgan in his 'Clinical Review' and was reproduced in journal articles over the following years, where it was used to illustrate the devastation syphilis could wreak on a family. Clearly, Morgan had spoken with members of the family in order to familiarize himself with the family history, and presumably the family trusted in his ability to treat them. The child was 'cured' by use of mercurial treatment after a failed series of inoculations.

Morgan did not entertain the possibility of a child contracting syphilis through sexual abuse or rape. He declared his position when he alluded to his support for fellow doctor William Wilde's assertions that among the poorest families, vaginal irritations caused by lack of hygiene in girls were sometimes mistaken for sexually transmitted diseases by inexperienced medical men who prescribed damaging mercurial treatment for them, leading to false accusations of rape.[56] This is the only allusion to sexual abuse within Morgan's work. In the case of one 8-year-old patient, Morgan noted without comment that she had stated 'that she was violated'.[57] The fact that Morgan gave no further details of the case suggests he had no wish to further the debate on abuse as it had no relevance to the treatment of his patient or his role as a medical man.[58]

Despite doctors' reluctance to comment on matters relating to children's sexuality, however they were infected, once hospitalized, girls' awareness of their sexuality marked them out as being morally as well as physically damaged.[59] Hospital governors and staff at the WLH constantly guarded against the hospital being used by older women to entice younger patients into prostitution. Morgan noted that the majority of patients were between the ages of 15 and 20, had recently become infected, and that the disease affected the young most virulently, 'soon reducing them from being specimens of youthful vigour, to the broken down aspect of sufferers from the syphilitic cachexia'.[60] He demonstrated his opinion of his female patients in a comment that also gave his prognosis for the long-term survival of children with syphilis:

> The syphilitic taint in the mother acts more potently, it would appear, than in the father – vast numbers of children die of this taint. Taking the patients under my care at the hospital this day, I find more than 50% of them have had children, of those who have as yet not been mothers, most of them are only a short time launched on a vicious life, and have casually escaped. Some of these have produced 3 and 4 children but out of these, but 2 have reached the ages of 7 and 9 years.[61]

In Morgan's view, whether they were sexually active within marriage or through prostitution, mothers were inherently responsible for the transmission of syphilis and the infection and death of their own children. The moral standing of mothers was of less importance at the WLH than at other hospitals when it came to the admission process. However, within the hospital itself those women who did not wish to be classed among 'street girls' in the common wards were obliged to demonstrate their respectability by producing a marriage certificate. This confirmed their moral respectability and differentiated them from common women in 'irregular unions' or the lowest class of patients.[62] It was important to women that this difference in their status be noted because of the stigma of sexual deviance attached to women with venereal disease. They were also extremely reluctant to have their infant stigmatized on account of the disease for which they were under treatment.[63] In other hospitals such women remained anathema. In 1854, female patients in the Richmond Hospital objected to poor syphilitic women being treated in the same hospital as them.[64] As late as 1889, the Board of Superintendence cautioned that admitting 'indiscriminately such patients into the wards of a General Hospital, and to associate them with women and children otherwise affected, would be highly objectionable'.[65] It is interesting to observe that women and children in this context were employed to symbolize innocence and respectability, diverging greatly from characterizations of the children of WLH patients.

CONCLUSIONS

A description of the symptoms of congenital syphilis suggests that the general condition of the child and its short life expectancy were at the root of the non-recording of infants at the WLH. The appearance of the disease and the disgust it engendered created a taboo within society, which even permeated the medical records of a hospital which specialized in treating syphilitic patients. Interest in pathologising sexually transmitted diseases made the government-funded WLH an ideal location for the observation and study of various forms of the disease and its appropriate treatments. As doctors recorded their observations of patients, child patients were instrumental in adding to the sum of knowledge of syphilis.

A distinct dichotomy arose in the treatment of syphilitic children. The immoral aura of sexual disease attached to the child and its visible lack of infant appeal caused tension for doctors whose professional instinct was their care and cure. Under Byrne's long tenure, children whose mothers repeatedly returned to the WLH had their cases followed with interest. Byrne paid close attention to their progress as the continued good health of the congenitally affected child was seen as a personal success for him.

In the mid-nineteenth century, the gendered discourse surrounding the CDA legislation created great hostility towards women with venereal disease and engendered societal perceptions of females as the locus of sexually transmitted disease. Although the CDA gave lock hospital doctors great control over their patients in Great Britain and in the Curragh, Cobh and Cork in Ireland, Dublin never came under their jurisdiction. Nonetheless, the hostility of the discourse surrounding the CDA permitted Morgan to use even young children for experimental trials. The WLH management's suspension of experimental inoculation brought respite to the patients, although the privacy of the hospital and its continued utility, rather than the comfort of patients or principles of consent to treatment, was central to the decision.

The question of culpability was also an important part of the mid-nineteenth-century discourse, focussing on the various means whereby children were infected by their diseased mothers. Little attention was paid to the likelihood of sexual abuse being the origin of infection in children, with doctors dismissing this possibility, emphasizing that the majority of the young girls at the WLH were over the age of 15 and were prostitutes. The stigmatization of children continued, however, as the harsh prognosis for the congenitally affected child and its pitiful appearance made it easy for it to be seen as the unfortunate by-product of sexual misalliance on the part of its parents. They were also perceived as examples of moral retribution, with the 'sins of the father' being visited on his offspring. It appears that syphilitic children were viewed pragmatically in the WLH, as part of the unfortunate sequelae of sexual disease, and as with their diseased mothers, they were deemed unacceptable in society and in medical discourse.

4

CHILDHOOD OPHTHALMIA IN IRISH WORKHOUSES, 1849–1861

Philomena Gorey

By 1849, physicians had identified ophthalmia as a specific disease with symptoms of inflammation of the conjunctiva or external coat of the eye. This inflammation commenced in the inside of the eyelid and, in many cases, extended to the globe of the eye – destroying the cornea or transparent coat, either by sloughing or subsequent ulceration, and producing complete or partial blindness in one or both eyes.[1] Contemporary medical authors linked the disease to poverty, overcrowding, monotonous diet, poor nutrition, exposure to cold and wet weather, inadequate clothing and bedding and lack of exercise, factors which, combined, contributed to poor general health and predisposition to the disease.[2] Ophthalmia was particularly omnipresent in mid-century Irish workhouses. It was prevalent especially in the months of June, July and August, and lessened in winter and spring. From 1847, during the distress of the Great Famine, when the hungry were crammed into workhouses as part of official relief strategies, there was a marked increase in the numbers presenting with the condition.[3] By 1849 it had come to official notice. The Poor Law Commissioners recorded that 'the prevalence of "sore eyes" and the appearance in some cases of a very severe type of ophthalmia was difficult to extirpate'.[4] By then the disease had reached epidemic proportions as wave after wave of outbreaks occurred simultaneously in workhouses throughout the midlands, south-west and west of Ireland. From then until the epidemic ended in 1853, a total 135,000 people contracted ophthalmia, with 95,000 being under the age of 15.[5]

The disease broke out in the Athlone Union Workhouse in April 1848, following instances in the town and surrounding countryside.[6] In Tipperary the outbreak was thought to have begun in the girls' schools in the town in autumn 1849.[7] The medical officer in the Limerick Union, Dr Kavanagh, reported that 2,000 cases had occurred in the workhouse, auxiliary workhouses and surrounding countryside between June and December 1850. In the south-west, George Huband, a Poor Law inspector in Cork, reported that ophthalmia was severe in the unions of Kanturk, Millstreet, Macroom, Dunmanway and Skibbereen, the main thoroughfare to the coast from County Limerick. The severity of the disease diminished further southward, meaning that the unions of Bantry, Castletownbere and Skull suffered little. It branched off at Kanturk, westward to Killarney and Kenmare, where the disease was very mild. The disease reached Cork city and Bandon by the main road from Macroom. In the west, the medical officers in Loughrea and Ballinasloe reported local epidemics. In Galway, Dr Brown reported a spread of the disease from the city workhouse to the two auxiliary workhouses, which were located in the country. Eastern locations were free of the epidemic.[8]

The severity and persistence of the epidemic prompted the Poor Law Commissioners to seek the assistance of Arthur Jacob and William Wilde. Jacob was Professor of Anatomy at the Royal College of Surgeons and surgeon for diseases of the eye at the City of Dublin Hospital.[9] He was an oculist who discovered the elements composing the layer of rod and cone cells in the retina of the eye; the so-called 'Jacob's Membrane'.[10] In 1839 he and Henry Maunsell founded the *Dublin Medical Press*, a weekly journal that campaigned for medical reform, and he remained as its editor

Figure 5. Towns where the Ophthalmia Epidemic was most severe.

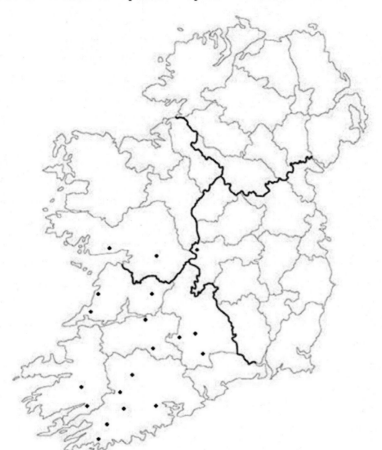

until 1859.[11] Wilde's interest in the eye stemmed from a period of practice at the Royal London Ophthalmic Hospital around 1823.[12] Following that, he travelled widely across Europe and the Middle East, where he witnessed trachoma or 'Egyptian Ophthalmia' at the military hospital first hand in Alexandria.[13] Wilde went to Vienna to improve his knowledge of ophthalmic and aural surgery at the *Allgemeines Krankenhaus*.[14] Upon returning to Dublin he founded St Mark's Hospital for Diseases of the Eye and Ear in 1844 and can be included as one of the leading players among the coterie of clinicians who pioneered the Dublin clinical school.[15] He held the position of editor of the *Dublin Quarterly Journal of Medical Science* between 1846 and 1849. The methodology that he applied to the collection of statistics on mortality and the status of disease, which also included the causes of handicap and sickness data in the censuses of 1841, 1851, 1861 and 1871, identify him as a competent statistician and this work was unsurpassed in contemporary Europe.[16] Jacob inspected the workhouse and auxiliary houses in Athlone in December 1849. Wilde went to the union schools, the workhouses and the ophthalmic hospital in Tipperary, followed by a further inspection in Athlone in August 1850. A lesser-known oculist, Dr M. Scraggs, spent the month of December 1851 at the Kanturk workhouse treating the patients there.[17] The task of the medical men was threefold. They were asked to inspect the accommodation at the workhouses, to examine the children in each union who had contracted ophthalmia, and to advise medical officers who had charge of the treatment and management of the epidemic.[18] This paper traces the progress of the epidemic, taking into account its two principal causes – nutritional deficiency and overcrowding. It examines the findings of the medical experts and the response of the Poor Law Commissioners, workhouse guardians and medical officers, who were all responsible for treating ophthalmia and managing the epidemic. Finally, it considers the ongoing care of those who had lost their sight and the provisions for the further development of their education and skills.

THE OPHTHALMIC OUTBREAK

The 1838 Poor Law (Ireland) Act provided for the establishment of workhouses for the relief of the destitute poor. The country was divided into 130 administrative areas, known as Poor Law Unions, which were funded by means of a property tax known as the poor rate. Relief was administered by boards of guardians, under the supervision and control of the English Poor Law Commission. Unlike England, relief would only be provided inside the workhouse, with no provision for outdoor relief. Relief was discretionary

Table 5. Incidence of Ophthalmia in Irish Workhouses, 1849-53

Year	Persons above 15 years		Children under 15 years of age		TOTAL	Cases arising in Workhouses	Cases with disease when admitted
	Male	Female	Male	Female			
1849	1,311	2,096	4,784	4,801	13,812*	11,368+	532+
1850	2,280	4,050	9,543	11,327	27,200	24,882	758
1851	3,670	6,821	14,252	18,370	45,947	42,067	963
1852	3,242	5,804	10,160	10,899	31,876	28,765	1,360
1853	1,594	3,660	4,614	6,009	16,013	14,555	1,291
Total	12,097	22,431	43,353	51,406	134,848	121,657	4,904

Source: *Fourth, fifth and sixth annual reports of the commissioners for administering the laws for relief of the poor in Ireland.*

*This total includes 820 cases from the Tipperary Union, which were not classified.

+The registry in several of the Unions does not distinguish whether the disease originated in or out of the Workhouse. The numbers in these two columns therefore do not correspond with the totals in the previous column.

and dependent on the availability of workhouse places.[19] As demonstrated in Table 5, the incidence of ophthalmia among children under 15 years of age vastly outnumbered that among persons aged over 15. In 1849, 932,284 people were admitted to workhouses and out of these 13,812 were medically treated for ophthalmia. In 1850, 27,200 of the 805,702 admitted presented with the disease.[20] The number of those infected peaked in 1851 with a high of almost 46,000 cases, and diminished in the following two years.[21] During the epidemic almost 95,000 children presented with ophthalmia.

The disease presented as a simple conjunctivitis. At this stage, inflammation occurred in the external part of the eye and the inside of the eyelids. This caused the eye to water and mucous to be discharged. These symptoms could be present among individual workhouse children for up to six months before an epidemic occurred. The medical officer of the Tipperary union, Dr Reardon, described the presenting cases as 'debilitated, starved, female children, generally those recently admitted, worn out by previous want and privations of every kind – many having refused to come into the house in consequence of its crowded state, until they were exhausted to the last degree'.[22] In the next stage of the disease, now at its most contagious, mucous or purulent discharge became abundant, and inflammation around the eye increased – closing the eye and swelling the upper lip, making it red in colour and globular in shape with a glossy surface. This swelling completely overlapped the lower lid. Ulceration of the cornea and protrusion of the iris of the eye followed, with the iris becoming adhered to the cornea. At this stage, the discharge was no longer a creamy matter but a thin red serum mixed with pus. Further ulceration to the membrane that lined the inside of the eyelid resulted in granulated or scar tissue – the so-called 'granular lids'. The great majority of cases that led to permanent, irreparable damage were at this chronic phase that proved less amenable to treatment. Chronic ophthalmia gave the transparent structures of the eye an opaque appearance and caused blindness.

Ophthalmia comprised conjunctivitis, catarrhal, purulent and gonorrhoeal ophthalmia and ophthalmia in the newborn. All were thought to be contagious. Purulent ophthalmia differed from other forms 'in the virulence of its contagion and the extreme rapidity of its course, rather than in any radical dissimilarity of nature'.[23] This was the form associated with overcrowding, where close contact with, and among, those affected was seen as the principal cause of ophthalmic epidemics. Outbreaks had previously been most common in army regiments and prisons. Around 1820, military authorities instructed the management of barracks to allow at least 500–800 cubic feet of air for each soldier. In the newly completed Mountjoy Gaol each prisoner was confined to a cell which measured 900 cubic feet.[24] However, a similar minimum standard of space for each individual was never fixed in the rules laid down for the instruction of Poor Law guardians. Instead, the matter was left to the discretion of boards. In 1847, the alarming spread of fever and dysentery in workhouses caused attention to be drawn to the matter of overcrowding. In their reports for that year, the Poor Law Commissioners warned guardians that limited workhouse space, an unwillingness to incur the expense of providing additional accommodation and persistence in admitting applicant after applicant – long after the limit of sanitary safety had been exceeded – ran the risk of creating high mortality by pestilence.[25]

In her case study of nutritional deficiency in Ireland in 1850, E. Margaret Crawford has illustrated how the form of ophthalmia prevalent during the Famine was a condition known as xerophthalmia, caused by lack of fat-soluble vitamin A and presented as dryness and ulceration of the cornea.[26] In view of the fact that contemporary accounts referred to the disease as ophthalmia, this paper will do likewise. By 1840, the potato had become the staple diet for the cottier and labouring classes – three-eighths of the population – with the average adult male estimated to consume between four and five kilos per day.[27] Although the potato was repeatedly castigated as a symbol of Irish poverty and economic backwardness, it was proven at the start of the Famine to be highly nutritious.[28] The one aspect missing from the nutritional value of the diet was vitamin A. Potatoes contain a negligible amount of the vitamin and in as much as whole milk is a good source of beta-carotene (the pro-vitamin of vitamin A), skimmed milk and buttermilk contain only very small amounts. Since both tended to be consumed instead of whole milk, for many the diet was practically devoid of the vitamin.[29] Crawford has analysed a dietary survey carried out by the Poor Law Commissioners in 1839 among the labourers of counties Limerick, Tipperary and Clare, and demonstrates the consumption of high values of protein, carbohydrates, calories and minerals, but grossly deficient vitamin A and vitamin D levels.[30] When potato blight, *phytophthora infestans*, caused failure of the crop in 1845 and subsequent years, and after the state abandoned its temporary soup kitchen scheme of 1847, workhouses became the last resort for those who depended on the potato as their only source of nourishment.

For dietary purposes, workhouse inmates fell into eight categories – able-bodied working males, able-bodied working females, those unable to work, children under 15 and over 9, boys under 9 and over 2, girls under 9 and over 2, infants under 2 and those convalescing in infirmary wards.[31]

Their diet largely consisted of oatmeal in stirabout – a form of porridge – potatoes and broth. Whole milk was given once a day; otherwise buttermilk or skimmed milk was supplied.[32] Meat, when included, was of poor quality. Diet was calculated to provide nourishment according to a general estimate of requirement with the least expense afforded and according to the circumstance of each union.[33] After the potato crop failed, the Commissioners authorized guardians to substitute potatoes for bread, soup or Indian corn meal.[34] The latter was an imported grain, principally from America, and was popular with workhouse guardians due to it being cheaper than oatmeal. Although initially unpopular, it became accepted as a dietary essential as other food sources became scarce. Many workhouses had financial difficulties, with guardians being hard pressed to honour contracts with suppliers.[35] Equally, a regular supply of milk proved difficult to procure, in many cases because of irregular payments to contractors. Lack of funds or supplies dictated that milk was, at times, substituted with cocoa, or a mixture made up of milk, water, rice and flour.[36]

MANAGEMENT AND TREATMENT

Medical officers were directly responsible for advising guardians on the numbers of applicants that could be admitted to workhouses without incurring the danger of disease. However, they could only recommend, and had no powers of enforcement. Furthermore, they were frequently the family attendants of the guardians as well as ratepayers, and their income may have been dependent on the same guardians. It was these officers who undertook the management of ophthalmia when it began spreading through workhouses and schools. Their first task was to separate those affected from the rest of the inmates. Suitable accommodation had to be procured for children and adults with the disease. Yet most people were unwilling to let their houses as hospitals, even at high rent. Consequently, old dilapidated dwellings, unoccupied mills, corn stores, breweries and other such buildings were rented by guardians out of necessity to act as temporary hospitals and auxiliary workhouses for the duration of the epidemic. Because of the ways in which these structures were formerly used, they were often located close to a river, meaning damp and wet conditions. Dr Reardon testified that the general health of the Tipperary workhouse:

> … was very bad indeed; we had cholera, dysentery, fever and small-pox, as well as several cases of gangrene and dropsy. There was no proper sewerage, neither was there sufficient water to cleanse the entire house or purify the privies, except what a horse brought daily from town.[37]

Between October 1849 and March 1850, 1,525 cases – 848 males and 677 females – of ophthalmia were treated in the Jail Lane Hospital in Tipperary before its closure following representations from the medical officers in favour of a larger building in Meeting House Lane, originally a corn store. However, one side of this building was without glazed windows, which made heating impossible. The four lofts it contained were converted into wards, each measuring eight and a half feet in height, but large beams that projected from each ceiling – placed there to support the heavy weight of corn – reduced the height of the ceilings, hence ventilation and lighting were inadequate.[38] Five hundred and forty-three cases were treated in Meeting House Lane and on the day of Wilde's inspection, 340 cases remained – 170 boys, 156 girls and 14 adults.

Wilde compiled a registry with the name, gender and age of the inmates, attaching observations to each entry with the intention of later drawing up a statistical statement on the condition of the disease in the workhouse generally and on the effects, and probable results, of the disease in each individual case. Rumours and discrepancies about the numbers becoming blind in unions were rife, and Wilde thought it right that the 'commissioners and guardians should distinctly understand the meaning to be attached to being "totally blind"', not least so that blame could not be unjustly levelled at medical officers.[39] He defined the 'totally blind' as those where 'both eyes had either become wasted and collapsed, or so much disorganised as to render all hope of vision irredeemable'.[40] On that basis he divided the patients into six classifications to stage the disease and facilitate the treatment:

> Class 1: All recent cases before they had passed into the chronic form. They should, where possible, be treated in the upper rooms of the house. Discharge from the eyes should be cleaned frequently with tepid water and a piece of tow – an inexpensive coarse part of flax – which should be thrown away immediately. He recommended that a number of adults could be instructed to carry out the procedure.
>
> Class 2: The irrevocably blind, who should be separated from the rest of the patients.
>
> Class 3: Those with ulcers of the cornea and protrusions of the iris or cornea, which did not produce loss of vision. In cases of protrusion of the cornea through the lids, which caused irritation, he recommended relieving the pressure of the fluid in the cornea by tapping the protruding part with a flat needle every now and then. In cases where the iris adhered to the cornea, he recommended the continued dilatation of the pupil with atropine.
>
> The first and third classes should be seen daily, the second class every third day.
>
> Class 4: Those with small, hard granulations, which were generally distinct and separate. These granulations should be touched every second day with sulphate of copper. 'Constitutional treatment' with bark or cod liver oil should be administered.
>
> Class 5: Those with large, hard, distinct granulations. Lids should be 'everted' every day by drawing the eyelid backwards against the orbit of the eye to expose the lining membrane of the upper lid and the granulations cut off with a curved scissors.[41] The inner surface of the lids could occasionally be scarified

slightly. Local astringents such as sulphate of copper, silver nitrate or acetate of lead should be applied as the granulations disappeared. Wilde recommended 'constitutional treatment' as in the previous class.

Class 6: Those in which the conjunctiva presented a uniform granular condition, with the surface of the granulations smooth. Ulceration of the cornea was usually present, which should be 'scarified' to relieve the pressure in the granulations and an application of finely ground acetate of lead should be used. The eye should then be washed with clean water, either by means of a syringe or sponge. The health of the patients was always run down, requiring as much meat as the diet of the institution permitted.[42]

For those with the more active form of the disease, Wilde recommended that swelling could be reduced with the application of 'a leech or two' to the local area, a procedure to be repeated daily. Cold applications to the eye and a solution of nitrate of silver to the lids were also thought to reduce swelling. He recommended, as soon as the swelling had subsided, everting the eyelid every day to examine the state of the conjunctival lining and to directly apply a solution of nitrate of silver so that granulated tissue would stop forming. If corneal ulcers had formed, they could be touched with the same solution with 'a fine camel's hair brush'. After doing this, atropine should be instilled into the eye to dilate the pupil. The eyelids were then to be closed with strips of adhesive, and lint, moistened with belladonna, placed over them and retained in position with a bandage. The eye was to remain shut for four days, but the lint was to be replaced if it became soiled with discharge. Because of crowded conditions, he recommended that patients be confined to bed. In mild chronic cases, which were the majority of cases he inspected (i.e. past the inflammation stage, with some granulated tissue but not blind), he suggested the use of wine of opium with an equal part of laurel water to be instilled into the eye daily. The average duration of the condition was thirty-five to forty days. Children spent approximately thirty days in workhouse infirmaries or temporary hospitals.[43]

THE EPIDEMIC IN DECLINE

By the time Jacob and Wilde inspected the Athlone facilities, the epidemic in the main workhouse appeared to be in decline, meaning that the precise numbers of cases was difficult to discern. One of two auxiliary workhouses was originally a malt house, located in a confined space near the river 'probably in order to facilitate the germination and fermentation process of the corn'.[44] This building had low vaults, narrow passages and tiny rooms considered unsuitable by Wilde for the maintenance of good health. He observed that many children in the girls' and boys' schools suffered from chronic ophthalmia, exhibiting growths in the lining membrane of the lids, but not ulcerated. He discussed their treatment with the medical officer, Dr O'Connell, advising him to inspect the children affected every five or six days at least, everting the eyelids to inspect the state of the conjunctiva and employing treatment according to the stage of the disease.

In March 1851 the Poor Law Commissioners dispersed a circular to inspectors in which they alluded to the strong evidence of skilful and successful treatment by medical officers. They pointed out that however great the value of professional skill might be in removing or alleviating the disease, guardians themselves were bound to use every precaution in their power to create an environment where patients could be treated, and to prevent, if possible, the spread of the disease. They stressed that two predisposing causes were the constitutional weakness of patients induced by famine and the necessity of lodging sufferers in wards, dormitories and day rooms while limiting their means of exercise to spaces enclosed by walls. The Commissioners pointed out that the general condition of the inmates was dependent on the will of the boards of guardians. They could improve health by ensuring ventilation of both dormitories and day rooms, sufficiency of clothing and bedding, varied food provisions, suitable employment and scrupulous attention to cleanliness.[45] Finally, they stressed that guardians had a duty to comply with the instructions of the medical officers for the classification and separate treatment of people with the acute and chronic forms of the disease and those who were convalescing. The Commissioners requested an immediate return of the numbers still affected in each facility.[46]

By this time the localities around the unions of Kanturk, Millstreet and Macroom appear to have been particularly stricken with ophthalmia, culminating in the epidemic spreading to the Kanturk workhouse. When afflicted paupers sought admission, the disease spread among the occupants, necessitating the acquisition of two additional auxiliary facilities – the Tan-Yard and the Quarry-House. As the names suggest, the Tan-Yard was situated on the edge of a river in the lowest part of town and the Quarry-House in a quarry-hole, the banks of which reached as high as the roof of the house on every side! This latter house was used as an ophthalmic hospital. Both were unfit for purpose. The medical officer, Dr Barry, reported that 2,051 females, 1,810 of whom were under 15, and 636 males, 352 under 15, had been treated for ophthalmia between October 1849 and 1851.[47] As few as 100 females and sixteen males lost the sight in one or both eyes. The guardians asked for the assistance of William Wilde, since the disease was still virulent. He refrained, but sent the aforementioned Dr Scraggs to oversee the treatment.

During the four weeks spent by Scraggs in the workhouse in December 1851, 130 ophthalmic patients were admitted to the workhouse, 120 of whom were children, the number of males and females being nearly equal. Scraggs found conditions in the main house good – the inmates well nourished and adequately clothed, and the building clean. One concern that emerged, however, was that patients were separated by gender rather than the medical classifications devised by Wilde. The disease was manageable, with most cases amenable to treatment and seldom proceeding to the dangerous stage.[48] By adhering rigidly to the principle of segregation, the numbers suffering from ophthalmia reduced from forty-six in the week of his first stay to seven during his last. The sight of all but two of the children was saved. One of those presented at the house in a chronic state and the other loss occurred in a boy who was convalescing but relapsed. On his departure he advised the guardians:

> Your duty, then, is simple: place your people as far as possible in circumstances approximating to their original condition as to space, by removing all unnecessary walls, sheds, &c.; provide extensive play-ground for your children; avoid keeping them too long confined in your crowded school and workrooms; enforce outdoor employment or exercise for all; do not overcrowd your dormitories; give up your Tan-Yard and Quarry-House auxiliaries as unfit for the residence of sick or well; provide others, if possible, in the countryside, which, I dare say, you can do equally cheap, and the saving will be considerable in medicine and doctoring; above all procure a suitable ophthalmic hospital, surrounded by a green field; require constant reports from your medical officer upon all sanitary matters; ask his opinion upon changes which you propose to make, particularly in reference to hospital arrangements; do all these, and you may expect to free yourselves from disease, mortality, and blindness; if you do not, you may be satisfied the present state of things must continue.[49]

A report in January 1852 penned by George Huband, the Poor Law inspector, vouched that improvements were being carried out in the workhouse. However, by the beginning of February, Dr Barry noted that 112 fresh cases had been treated by him.[50] A medical inspector, Dr Purcell, confirmed that a mild form of the disease had recurred. He attributed this to overcrowding in the female side of the house. The women's spinning room held 440 women, and contained 30,545 cubic feet of air, which allowed 70 cubic feet per person – well below the recommended 500 cubic feet per person. The girl's schoolroom was almost half the size, contained 305 children and 16,194 cubic feet of air, which allowed 54 cubic feet for each child. At 2 p.m.

each day, 64 additional children came into it from the embroidery school, which reduced the quantity to 42 cubic feet of air for each child.[51] In spite of this, virulent ophthalmia did not return to the workhouse and numbers continued to fall very gradually.

At the time of the inspections children were accommodated in three facilities in Athlone, four in Tipperary and three in Kanturk. The numbers of children in each house varied between 250 and 400 children. Segregation into acute, chronic and convalescing cases demanded that children were constantly being moved from one facility to another depending on the stage of their disease or on the need for the weaker children to be in a more comfortable environment. Throughout the epidemic, there was never adequate space or healthy, warm locations to accommodate all children at the same time. As soon as the dangerous acute phase of the disease passed, children were moved on to inferior quarters to make room for the next group. This meant there was always a fear that convalescing children would relapse.

Why should ophthalmia have been more prevalent in these particular regions and their local workhouses and why were children more likely to succumb to the disease than adults? Ó Gráda and Mokyr point to a number of famine conditions that greatly increased the susceptibility of the body to disease as resistance declined. The impact of malnourishment led to a decline in physical energy output, the consequence of which was that activities such as the ability to work or to look after a household suffered. Families left their homes in search of food, leaving behind the facilities for maintaining the basic requirements for daily living like cooking and hygiene. The epidemic occurred after sustained periods of poor nutrition, resulting in a fall in essential vitamins, in this case vitamin A.[52] All of these conditions were present among workhouse children. A combination of poor general health, overcrowding and inadequate facilities for the treatment of childhood illness contributed to ophthalmic outbreaks. The greatest hazard to recovery lay in the inability of guardians to provide suitable temporary treatment centres, whether due to a lack of funds, a belief that the epidemic would dissipate in a short time or a view that spending money on furnishing temporary facilities was wasteful. Ophthalmia was not a fatal disease. Unlike cholera, typhoid or dysentery, mortality among those who contracted it was negligible, so the same urgency to eliminate it did not prevail.[53] Furthermore, the epidemic occurred towards the end of the period of distress. By this time, the Commissioners of Health, who had been appointed to oversee the management of disease during the Famine, had concluded that temporary hospitals had been erected in greater numbers than would have been sufficient and expenses were thus incurred that could have been avoided.[54] Once children were admitted into the workhouses, the pressure for space dictated the practice of placing several children in a bed together at night. Along with this, they were congregated together into closed schoolrooms during the day.[55] These circumstances go some way towards explaining why children were more susceptible to ophthalmia than adults. Most children, however, did recover without full loss of sight. Granular lids were the chief cause of impaired vision and blindness.

CONCLUSIONS

Although the Famine has long been associated with mass death and the spread of epidemic diseases, it is easy to forget that the health of children who survived was often severely impaired. Although fortunate enough to escape death, an important and often understated legacy of the Famine was that the generation who grew up in the following decades was at a physical disadvantage. Wilde had warned that blind people live long lives and that chronic ophthalmia sometimes rendered sufferers incapable of earning their own livelihood, and, in some cases, of ever leaving the workhouse.[56] By the mid-1850s, a debate had begun as to the further care of the visually impaired. In 1857 there were 796 blind people accommodated in workhouses who had lost their sight as a direct result of disease during the Famine. This accounted for 0.48 per cent, or one in 200 of the 166,342 treated for ophthalmia in the workhouses, but did not include those who were treated and lost their sight outside the facilities.[57] The question arose as to the extent to which accommodation specially adapted to their maintenance should be provided at the expense of the poor rate. There were nine blind asylums in Ireland at this time, where residents could learn a range of subjects and skills.[58] The Poor Law Commissioners did not necessarily agree with isolating the blind from 'the outward world' in these institutions, but these facilities presented an opportunity for industrial teaching of the young 'for a limited time to acquire the means of wholly or partially maintaining themselves'.[59] John Blake, MP for Waterford, took up the cause of the blind, calling attention to the age restriction of 22 years for admission to an asylum. He and others hoped that the government would consent to the withdrawal of the age limit in the preamble to the Poor Relief (Ireland) Bill before parliament at the time.[60] Blake's cause did not succeed on two grounds in particular. One was the belief that blind individuals who had not been educated before their twenties had little hope of learning new skills. The other was because withdrawal of the age limit would require an extension of accommodation in the asylums, which at the time comprised 440 places. Educational opportunities for Famine victims were lost, many of whom would have been in their twenties by the time the Poor Relief Act of 1862 was passed. The age restriction for admission to blind asylums for the workhouse blind was eventually lifted in 1878 provided that the 'reception, maintenance and instruction of every pauper not exceed the sum of five shillings weekly'.[61]

Ophthalmia had long been associated with poverty and overcrowding. Although Famine conditions emphasized the high risk and incidence of the disease, it did not affect or advance medical knowledge. Wilde's treatments were not new. Silver nitrate and copper sulphate were among the pharmacopeia of preparations used to treat the disease in the mid-nineteenth century. Segregation of those inflicted was recognized as a first step in the prevention of contagion. Wilde and Jacob were among the last ophthalmologists who did not have the benefit of the ophthalmoscope.

In 1851, Hermann von Helmholtz developed the instrument, which was to revolutionize the progress of ophthalmology. Prior to his invention, ophthalmologists could not view the back of the eye and struggled to explain certain classes of eye disease in which there was loss of vision.[62] The ophthalmoscope allowed medical men to look inside the living eye, to recognize and accurately describe the differing diseases of, for example, the optic nerve and the retina and their connection with the brain and other organs, thus establishing scientific principles and connecting the eye more closely with general medicine.

5

CHILDREN AND THE FALLING SICKNESS, IRELAND, 1850–1904

June Cooper

*H*istorical accounts of epilepsy have been primarily a story of adult experience. In the Irish context, while historians have devoted some attention to the care of children with intellectual disabilities,[1] far less has been said about epilepsy. During the period under review here (1850–1904), paediatric epilepsy was treated according to the age, extent and character of the disorder in individual cases: the severity and frequency of seizures determined the stage at which medical intervention was deemed necessary. Parents played a pivotal role in securing medical relief for their children. The method and means of treatment was influenced by therapeutic and scientific advances and modern neurology. In addition, the perceived and actual psychiatric manifestations of the condition informed treatment choices. However, did these interconnected approaches specifically treat the 'epileptic' child? This chapter firstly examines the general recommendations for the medical treatment of epilepsy, and the development of treatment by drugs in Ireland. Where possible, it indicates whether medical care was child orientated, and whether medical intervention healed or harmed.

Secondly, it examines the institutional treatment of chronic cases – children who were diagnosed with psychiatric or other complications. Using the Richmond District Lunatic Asylum as a case study, it seeks to understand the justifications for committing these children to lunatic asylums with predominately adult insane populations, and analyses their medical care while confined, and the long-term outcomes for those admitted.

The Richmond District Lunatic Asylum collection contains limited, yet extremely rich, source material relating to epilepsy in childhood. Medical casebooks, both male and female, admission registers, and minutes of committee meetings have been examined. Additional sources used in this study include contemporary medical journals, medical textbooks, and parliamentary papers.

ROBERT J. GRAVES AND ROBERT BENTLEY TODD

To begin with, it is necessary to introduce two highly influential Irish doctors who contributed to the development of epilepsy treatments in Ireland. Robert J. Graves, physician to the Meath Hospital from 1821 to 1843, provided invaluable observations on epilepsy and treatment advice in clinical lectures and medical journal papers. He is also recognized as the first to describe peripheral neuritis.[2] Examples of his many other achievements include bringing the stethoscope to Ireland, 'feeding fevers',[3] the identification of 'exophthalmic goitre' (thereafter known as Graves' disease), and his bedside clinical teaching methods, which became world renowned.[4]

Robert Bentley Todd has been described as 'one of the first precursor-neurologists'.[5] Born in Dublin, Todd later became Dr Graves' student. He was a resident of London by 1830, became licentiate of the Royal College of Surgeons in Ireland in 1831, and co-founded the King's College Hospital, London in 1840.[6] In his Lumleian Lectures, 1849, Todd described 'post-ictal' paralysis, known as Todd's paralysis, and presented a neurophysiological theory that paved the way for modern neurologists.[7] He later confirmed that convulsions during dentition indicated a susceptibility to the onset of epilepsy in later years.[8] Apart from nervous diseases, he also contributed to the study of febrile illnesses and liver disease.[9]

TREATING THE 'EPILEPTIC' CHILD

Doctors recognized that children were prone to develop epilepsy at dentition, primary and secondary, and puberty.[10] Convulsions in infancy and childhood accounted for high rates of infant and child mortality in Ireland. A clear distinction was not made between deaths due to convulsions and deaths due to epilepsy.[11] Therefore, the incidence of epilepsy was not accurately documented. Generally, medical intervention or constant medical care was not necessarily a requirement for older children unless the number, duration and severity of seizures increased,[12] or the seizures changed in character. *Grand mal* referred to convulsive, *petit mal* to non-convulsive 'attacks'.[13] In the case of *grand mal*, the action of falling, the potential for choking and suffocation were all potentially life-threatening without due care from parents.[14] The recurrence of seizures varied from once a day or week to once a year.[15] It was recognized that epilepsy, as opposed to childhood convulsions, 'usually assumes a periodic character in children'.[16] Children may not have received any medical assistance until their health had deteriorated significantly and they were dependent on their guardians to seek medical relief on their behalf.

The sick poor received medical care in workhouse infirmaries, voluntary hospitals, dispensaries and in their own home. The dispensary system was improved considerably under the terms of the 1851 Medical Charities (Ireland) Act.[17] However, despite these reforms, medical assistance was not automatically available to, or sought by, the sick poor.[18] Apart from orthodox medicine, they may have had recourse to traditional herbal medicine which was practised particularly in rural areas.[19]

Homoeopathy, which was supported mainly by the better off, also had a limited presence. By 1850 its formal organization had taken place in Dublin.[20] The voluntary-funded Dublin Homoeopathic Institute and Dispensary opened in 1844; the Irish Homoeopathic Society was set up in April 1845;[21] and the Belfast Dispensary was founded on 1 August 1848.[22]

Sir William Wilde, a highly influential aural and ophthalmic surgeon at St Mark's Ophthalmic Hospital, acknowledged that homoeopathy, which used infinitesimal doses of medicine, condemned blood-letting and purgative medicine for children,[23] had curbed the general orthodox tendency to prescribe heroic doses.[24]

In the 1850s the recommended course of orthodox medical treatment for epilepsy comprised three parts, the core of which remained unchanged: prophylactic measures, care during and after seizures, particularly *grand mal*, and attempts to reduce further attacks. The general medical advice in paediatric cases depended on age and constitution. It included lancing of gums during dentition,[25] a change of air between 'fits' which 'proves of especial benefit in the cases of children',[26] a quiet, darkened room, plenty of rest, and attention to a light but nutritious diet.[27] Arrowroot, which was considered particularly suitable for infants and young children and usually prepared with milk and flavoured with lemon or sugar,[28] was given after 'fits'.[29] In addition, doctors attempted to remove all exciting causes or 'irritations', for example intestinal worms and constipation, to prevent further attacks.[30] Purgative medicine such as turpentine, specifically for tapeworms,[31] and calomel, a milder laxative, was advised for children, if strong.[32] Generally, graduated doses of medicine were recommended depending on the child's age,[33] although it is worth noting that the child was likely to have struggled against its administration in any form.[34] A combination of scammony, white sugar and calomel was considered suitable for children because it tasted and smelled the same as 'rich new milk'.[35] Sulphate of copper, an antispasmodic, was suggested for patients who had developed epilepsy at puberty.[36] Not all doctors followed these instructions. The quality of medical care depended on a number of factors including the calibre of the doctor – up until the 1858 Medical Registration Act, qualification requirements for dispensary doctors were not standardized.[37] Other common issues included a lack of familiarity with, and understanding of, epilepsy, such as new theories and treatments, and the suitable care of children.

Blood-letting was usually resorted to in cases of suspected cerebral congestion, which may have occurred following a succession of severe 'fits', and only if the patient was not 'weak or irritable'.[38] There is evidence that, in certain cases, children were treated by the following method into the 1860s:[39] the head was shaved, leeches were applied, the neck blistered and purgative medicine administered.[40] The condition was thought to be serious enough to warrant such intervention.[41] However, doctors differed in opinion as to its potential risks.[42] In 1852 a mother brought her 5-year-old son – who suffered from 'fits' at dentition, which subsequently 'merged into regular epilepsy' following a series of attacks[43] – to the South Dublin Union Hospital, the workhouse infirmary, where he was treated by this method. Days later he died.[44] In other cases older children, or those who were likely to have been more robust, recovered fully after the treatment.[45]

Eager to find a cure, doctors in Ireland and elsewhere regularly promoted novel anti-epileptic remedies. In the 1840s Wilde[46] promoted traditional Irish herbal remedies in order to promote a 'distinctive school of Irish medicine'.[47] He had developed an enthusiasm for Irish folklore as a child in the west of Ireland.[48] In the 1840s and 1850s herbal remedies were increasingly cited as adjuncts to, rather than replacements for, purgative medicine, dietetics, and change of air. In 1845, the esteemed Dr Dominic Corrigan, physician to the House of Industry Hospitals, recorded his findings on digitalis. *Digitalis purpurea*, or Lus Mór in Irish, was a traditional Irish herbal remedy that was prepared from foxglove leaves. Corrigan reported its 'quack' origins and its effectiveness when administered in regulated doses.[49] The 'herb woman' or 'fairy-doctress'[50] believed that 'epileptic' children had been seized by fairies; that digitalis would kill the fairies thereby enabling the children's return.[51] In some cases children were given fatal doses.[52] In 1852, Graves recommended the long-known Irish cure, *cotyledon umbilicus*, which was also used to treat asthma.[53] He noted the case of a 4-year-old boy who was cured by the remedy.[54] Dr Jonathon Osborne, King's Professor of Materia Medica, physician to Mercer's Hospital, Dublin, restated the positive action of digitalis in 1856.[55] The intersection of orthodox and unorthodox medicine through the influence of homoeopathy and the inclusion of Irish herbal remedies, which perhaps normalized orthodox medicine to those who would have otherwise rejected it, was a positive development in the treatment of paediatric epilepsy.

However, bromide of potassium, hailed as the first effective anti-epileptic drug, was the most significant addition to the therapeutic gamut.[56] Sir Charles Locock advocated its use in the treatment of epilepsy in 1857. Dr J.M. Purser, physician to the Whitworth Hospital, Drumcondra and Demonstrator of Anatomy in the Carmichael School of Medicine, carried out experiments to ensure its safety and effectiveness in the treatment of epilepsy. His paper, published in 1869, confirmed its efficacy; however, he indicated its potentially harmful effects on the respiratory system, the heart and the skin,[57] and mental dullness, also known as bromism, when administered in excessive doses.[58] Purser's important work served as an excellent guide to the medical profession. The following year, Dr Walter Smith, Senior Demonstrator of Anatomy in the School of Physic and assistant physician to the Adelaide Hospital, reported that bromide of potassium[59] was used by doctors in France as a sedative for young children in cases of 'wakefulness' but that it should not be given to children with diarrhoea.[60] He also remarked that one ton was produced in England weekly for medicinal use and stressed that the drug had been found to exacerbate epilepsy in cases of 'cerebral and spinal anaemia'.[61] Dr Thomas Hayden, physician to the Mater Misericordiae Hospital, reported positive results in his trials on adult patients and recommended its use in lunatic asylums.[62] Despite numerous cautionary reports regarding its secondary effects, primarily in relation to heroic doses,[63] according to other doctors the medicine delayed seizures for months and in some cases years.[64] The benefits of successfully controlling seizures were thought to outweigh any of the unpleasant side effects. Bromide of potassium was administered to children with epilepsy in Ireland.[65] If the drug rendered a 'cure', which was often temporary, only minimal medical care was needed.

MODERN NEUROLOGY AND PSYCHIATRY

The National Hospital for the Relief and Cure of the Paralysed and Epileptic in London was established in 1860. It was at the National Hospital, Queen

Square that John Hughlings Jackson, William Richard Gowers, John Russell Reynolds and Edward Henry Sieveking built upon the legacies of Todd, among a host of others. The formulation of a clear definition of the aetiology and nosology of epilepsy was the most important starting point from which further study could develop.[66] Jackson, referred to as the pioneer of modern neurology, defined epilepsy as the 'occasional, sudden, excessive, rapid, and local discharge of grey matter'[67] in 1873, subsequently noting it as a chronic disorder.[68] Jackson's definition was heavily influenced by Todd's earlier theories.[69] In the last decades of the nineteenth century, brain injury and epilepsy were increasingly linked.[70] In some cases, Irish doctors traced its origin to paediatric meningitis.[71] Scientific advances such as anaesthetics, anti-septic surgery and the introduction of the X-ray in 1895 by Wilhelm Roentgen facilitated progress in epileptology. Neurosurgery was performed by Sir Charles Ball, University Examiner in Surgery, and Surgeon to Sir Patrick Dun's Hospital, in the late nineteenth century.[72] However, modern neurology was a work in progress and its impact was not immediate. Moreover, there was another crucial aspect to the debate on epilepsy – the influence of psychiatry.

In the nineteenth century the lines between epilepsy and insanity were blurred, and 'epileptics' were frequently committed to lunatic asylums. Resident physicians of lunatic asylums observed large numbers of patients with the disorder and played a key role in defining contemporary interpretations of epilepsy. For example, in the 1830s, Esquirol recorded masturbation as a secondary cause of the disorder; a theory disputed by neurologists such as Gowers in the 1880s, who viewed it as a consequence, not a cause.[73] Thus, from the 1860s, there was an ongoing neuropsychiatric debate on epilepsy. Patterns of the hereditary character of insanity were also observed in lunatic asylums and came under ever-increasing scrutiny. French alienist Benedict Augustin Morel, and Henry Maudsley, resident physician of the Manchester Royal Lunatic Asylum, a leading British alienist and editor of the *British Journal of Mental Science*,[74] were central figures in the popularization of the degeneration theory in the second half of the nineteenth century. Epilepsy in a parent was thought to produce other forms of insanity in the child.[75] In the 1870s Cesere Lombrosso associated epilepsy with criminality.[76] Dementia praecox or schizophrenia in young people was considered part of the final stages of degeneration.[77] During the *fin-de-siècle* period, there were grave concerns about the apparent rise of insanity, degeneration and the wider debate on national decline.[78] Links between insanity, epilepsy and mental impairment were reinforced by the eugenics movement of the early twentieth century, placing sufferers in a most vulnerable position.[79]

INSTITUTIONAL TREATMENT

An expansive state-funded asylum system for the insane was developed in Ireland in the first half of the nineteenth century. In 1843 sufferers of epilepsy, 'where the fits produce imbecility of mind as well as body',[80] were deemed eligible for admission to lunatic asylums. Nevertheless, due to limited asylum accommodation, workhouses were recommended as an alternative; the decision to do so was based largely on a lack of public finances.[81] Children with epilepsy became inmates of workhouses throughout the period. While Joseph Lalor, resident physician at Richmond District Lunatic Asylum from 1858 to 1886, was sympathetic to the plight of 'incurables', he nevertheless opposed their admission because precious beds for curable patients were forfeited in the process.[82] Workhouse guardians were equally opposed to the admission of 'curable or incurable' lunatics, 'no suitable staff being maintained for their proper treatment'.[83] 'Epileptics', particularly chronic cases, were unwanted in workhouses and lunatic asylums because neither could provide adequate care.

According to the Richmond admission registers, it was not until after 1867 and the introduction of the Dangerous Lunatics Act (1867)[84] that child admissions increased. A general rise in committal numbers following the act led to concerns that the system was being abused. In 1872 an inspector of lunacy suggested that 'even children when troublesome, noisy, difficult to control or idiotic are constantly drafted off to District Asylums as dangerous' (dangerous referred more to the criminal context).[85] It was incumbent on dispensary doctors to certify the committals. Children were transferred from workhouses and private residences in relatively equal measure. In the case of the Richmond, one child was admitted in 1867, four children were admitted in 1868, and nine children with a variety of disorders in 1869. From 1869 onwards, two children with epilepsy were admitted on average annually.[86] However, these figures may not be conclusive. Children's 'mental condition' and the cause of insanity were recorded in the admission registers, though the cause of insanity was not always noted. Therefore, children admitted with, for instance, mania could have been suffering from epilepsy but this fact may not have been reported in the register. The average age of children on admission was 13 years, although in a minor number of cases children were aged as young as 5.

The duration of the 'attacks' prior to the children's admission ranged from four days to a period of months. However, for the most part, children suffered from epilepsy for a number of years prior to their admission to the Richmond.[87] This suggests that their condition had worsened over a period of time until their confinement became necessary because they required greater medical care, or were viewed as a burden on the workhouse. It is also probable that some parents sent their children to district asylums because they were regarded as a source of shame. In 1879, inspector of reformatory and industrial schools John Lentaigne stressed that his attempts to admit 'epileptic' children were hindered by the school managers, who 'generally entertain such an exaggerated dread of the disease'.[88] The practicalities of caring for children requiring constant supervision perhaps also became too great. In 1891, the inspectors of lunacy in Ireland reported that a mother in Dublin chained her 'imbecile child' to her bedstead daily because she had no one to care for him while she went out to work.[89]

The five headings under which children with epilepsy were most frequently admitted to the Richmond were 'suicidal', 'dementia', 'mania', 'imbecile' and 'congenital epilepsy'. To threaten or attempt suicide was viewed as insanity.[90] Mania was also recognized as a form of insanity. 'Epileptic imbecile' described those whose 'mental function' was thought to have diminished as a result of their condition.[91] In 1839 Graves referred to the case of a young boy who endured ten 'fits' daily for six years and 'lapsed into idiotcy'.[92] Todd warned that epilepsy was likely to produce 'dementia or other forms of insanity'[93] and that repeated *petit mal* seizures were 'in general pretty certain precursors of a state of dementia or fatuity'.[94] The Stewart Institute for Training and Educating Idiotic and Imbecile Children, which was founded by Henry Hutchinson Stewart and George Kidd in 1869, received requests from a special committee in 1870 to set up an epileptic ward 'on the pleas that the two conditions, idiocy and epilepsy, are very closely associated'.[95] Stewart's approved the request and a fund was started.[96] Epilepsy was considered a cause of mental impairment and was occasionally cited in the Richmond admission registers as a cause of 'idiocy'.

The moral treatment system initiated at the Richmond by Lalor, which focused on recreation, work, education and the happiness of its patients, stood out at a time of pessimism over the curative ability of lunatic asylums.[97] Lalor, who was influenced by John Connolly and the non-restraint movement,[98] endeavoured to reduce physical restraint in any form.[99] Evidence from medical casebooks suggests that 'epileptic' patients were regularly placed in seclusion because they became 'very excited' and violent prior to or after 'fits'. While in seclusion, a female patient, whose age was not given, 'destroyed several pairs of blankets, sheets, and also her own clothes'.[100] Diet and fresh air were the main means by which doctors in asylums could care for patients, particularly those who were bedridden.[101] In the 1870s and 1880s sedatives were increasingly prescribed.[102] Dr Connolly Norman, appointed medical superintendent of the Richmond following Lalor's death, prescribed sulphonal for over a decade. It was subsequently ascertained that the drug caused serious kidney damage.[103] As discussed earlier, bromide of potassium was the primary anti-epileptic drug in use at this time. Questions were also raised about its long-term effects. In 1899 Norman refuted claims that bromide of potassium caused chronic 'epileptics' to become demented; he stated that the allegations were 'exaggerated' and 'demonstrably untrue in the majority of cases'.[104] In doing so, he accepted the validity of the claim in a minority of cases.

By the late nineteenth century, children continued to languish in workhouses with little medical care. For example, the inspectors of lunacy reported in 1891 that 'an epileptic child aged eight with congenital weakness of one side, although she could walk well, was for a great part of each day in bed because she was troublesome and destructive, and has never been in the open air since May 1886'.[105] In 1895 nuns were enlisted as nurses in a number of workhouse hospitals, which replaced the old system whereby fellow workhouse inmates provided care.[106] The 1899 Elementary Education (Defective and Epileptic Children) Act, which enabled the foundation of special schools and classes, was not introduced in Ireland.[107] Following the 1898 Local Government Act, district asylums became the responsibility of county councils.[108] At the close of 1880, there were 1,022 patients and 72 vacancies at the Richmond.[109] By 1892 there were approximately 1,500 patients.[110] Due to such overcrowding, the decision was made to build an auxiliary to the Richmond. The Portrane asylum was originally intended for chronic cases; however, it was eventually constructed to accommodate 1,200 of all classes.[111] Norman, who favoured the system of boarding out the insane over institutional care, said of chronic patients that 'such people require constant medical attention and assiduous nursing'.[112] Beginning in 1902, 'epileptics' and 'congenital mental defectives' from the Richmond were transferred to Portrane. Large numbers of workhouse inmates were also transferred to asylums at this time.[113]

Two cases selected from the late nineteenth and early twentieth century illustrate the extended confinement of children with epilepsy, and medical observations of their cases. Although the first case documents the medical treatment of the patient primarily in his adult years, it nonetheless provides insights into the chronic nature of the disorder in individual cases and traces the life of a child following admission to the asylum. In 1886, a 13-year-old 'school boy' was admitted as a dangerous lunatic to the Richmond. His mental condition on admission was reported as suicidal dementia. In 1898, twelve years later, work on a retrospective medical casebook began. The first entry recalls the patient's case history from the time of his admission in 1886 to 1898. It noted that 'he has had a habit of picking up old bits of steel and made an attempt on the life of another patient by jumping up on his back unawares and cutting his throat with a piece of steel. He also attempted to tear the eyes out of a patient. Masturbates excessively'.[114] The next entry described his mental and physical health in 1898, then a 25-year-old man. His decaying teeth, his well-nourished body, and his soft but regular pulse were noted; his lungs, heart and abdomen were also examined.

His mental condition was described as 'altogether very childlike in manner'.[115] A 'chart of periodical events' was started in 1898 to record seizure frequency. The patient's weight was also monitored. In April 1899 an unspecified dosage of potassium bromide was administered. In October 1899 the medical officer documented the patient's response to a brief period of respite: 'thanks be to God I am well, I never have a fit now, I think they are all gone'.[116] A subsequent entry in April 1900 stated that he had six severe fits but that 'he will not take medicine'.[117] In a period of less than six months, from April to October 1901, he had endured '103 fits by day and 33 by night'.[118] From November 1901 to early April 1902 he suffered 131 seizures and 'hears voices'.[119] His weight dropped considerably after a succession of 'fits'. During periods of increased seizure frequency, he was transferred to division five – the male infirmary. The patient regularly inquired about his relatives and their infrequent visits and was acutely aware of his protracted stay in the asylum.[120] He was recorded as having a good appetite, sleeping well and being in good general physical health. He was transferred to Portrane in 1902 and died there in 1913 aged 40.

In October 1903 a 6-year-old boy was admitted to the Richmond as a 'congenital mental defective' with hereditary epilepsy. He was recorded as 'completely imbecile'. His family medical history showed a predisposition for 'mental defect'. The patient fell when two and a half years of age and was in convulsions for six hours afterwards. He had suffered three 'epileptic fits' after sunstroke. He was described as 'dirty, makes a crowing noise but does not speak, does not give active trouble, is restless, runs about the ward laughing and crowing'.[121] A subsequent entry stated that 'he had been heard to say dada but nothing else, restless'.[122] In April the medical officer reported that the child's right arm was 'wasted and no growth for some time past'.[123] In June 1904, a nurse observed that 'he has had occasional little weaknesses during the last two weeks, that is he falls back in a chair in a kind of faint and seems quite unconscious for all of a minute then quietly gets right again'.[124] He was later reported as suffering from 'frequent attacks of petit mal'.[125] In 1907 the medical officer stated that he 'does not appear to understand anything that is said to him – appetite and sleep good'.[126] One year later he was described as 'noisy, restless, can't keep quiet for a moment. Had two fits three months ago.'[127] The type of 'fit', whether *petit* or *grand mal*, was not documented. This boy's record was found in the female medical casebook. He was kept in the female ward due to his age. He was said 'to show affection to the patient who looks after him'.[128] He was subsequently transferred to the male ward in 1909. He died in February 1910; no cause of death was given.

In both cases records were kept of seizure frequency. (In the 1850s seizures were not recorded at the Richmond.)[129] In the first case the patients' seizures were documented systematically, and he was examined by a medical officer at least twice a year. Despite a reduction in seizures following medication, the patient subsequently refused to take it, which raises questions about the true extent of its side effects. In the second case, the decision to leave the boy in the female ward showed concern for his age. The nurse's identification of his 'little weaknesses', and the problems with his arm, indicate that he was relatively closely monitored. Children were initially reported on weekly, then monthly. By the end of the nineteenth century heredity was considered the leading cause of insanity.[130] For a number of years, the Richmond had stated the familial relationships of patients in the asylum and the hereditary nature of insanity in its annual reports.[131] A final example from the Richmond medical casebooks illustrates the extent to which entire families were affected by epilepsy. A girl aged 9 was admitted to the asylum from the workhouse as a congenital mental defective with suspected epilepsy in 1903. The medical casebook stated that she was 'subject to sudden unaccountable fits of very violent passion';[132] the term epilepsy was not used. She was 'quite blind'. She asked when she could go to find her mother, explaining that her mother was in 'some institution'. Unbeknown to the girl, her mother, who suffered from epilepsy, was also a patient at the Richmond. The little girl was placed in division twenty-two, her mother in division eleven.[133] It seems likely that her mother's condition and the child's 'destructive behaviour', which was referred to in the medical casebook, were catalysts for her committal. Her mother's case file states: 'daughter inmate of North Dublin Union – blind, epileptic, imbecile'.[134] The girl was transferred to Portrane, where she died in 1930. Her mother died at the Richmond in 1913.[135]

The Royal Commission on the Care and Control of the Feeble-minded was set up in 1904. It was said that in Ireland 'epilepsy was regarded as more of a family disgrace than was insanity'.[136] Most of the children who were admitted to the Richmond with epilepsy died there following periods of between one and seven years. A minor number were discharged as 'relieved'. In a small number of cases patients had been confined in the Richmond and Portrane for a total of eighteen to twenty-one years.

CONCLUSIONS

The degree and type of medical care required for children with epilepsy in the second half of the nineteenth century was dependent on age of onset and the severity of the condition in individual cases. Manageable symptoms did not necessitate constant medical attention. Infant and child mortality rates due to convulsions remained high. According to statistical records, from 1886 to 1896, 'convulsions' accounted for 20,764 infant deaths and the deaths of 25,261 under-5s. During the same period, twenty infants and sixty-five under-5s died from epilepsy.[137] As in previous decades, these figures could not be relied upon because the primary cause of the 'convulsions' was not always documented.[138] Such ambiguity was attributed to the absence of medical attendance, and therefore diagnosis, in numerous cases.[139] Inadequate medical training in the field of children's diseases was also thought responsible.[140] Children's access to medical relief depended on its availability, parental responses to the illness and their preference for orthodox or unorthodox medicine.

For most of the period under review, workhouses provided little medical care for children with epilepsy and they were transferred to district asylums where possible. Parents were likely to have sent their children to asylums because of stigma, to receive medical care, because adverse social circumstances occasioned it or for a combination of all three motivations. A specialized institution was not founded for chronic cases in Ireland. However, the establishment of the Portrane auxiliary was a crucial alternative. While the dangers of the asylum were many – they were defenceless children surrounded by adults, many of whom were violent and unpredictable – they were at least better placed in respect of access to medical assistance than workhouses or in neglectful family homes. Children's lives were undoubtedly prolonged as a result of their committal. Nevertheless, the sense of cessation of time following admission, as poignantly described by Mark Finnane,[141] is even more palpable in the case of children, a small number of whom grew up in the Richmond and died at Portrane.

6

CONSTRUCTING 'MORAL HOSPITALS': IMPROVING BODIES AND MINDS IN IRISH REFORMATORIES AND INDUSTRIAL SCHOOLS, C. 1851–1890

Ian Miller

*I*n 1851 the inspectors-general of Irish prisons proclaimed that 25 per cent of petty larceny cases brought to trial in Dublin over the previous year had involved youths who had migrated to the city during the Famine. Forced to survive without the positive moral influence of parental guidance, many of the 'destitute and friendless orphans of those who fell victim to the famine' were portrayed as having fallen into the company of older prison offenders who taught them how to pickpocket and steal.[1] Although anxieties about rising levels of juvenile criminality were common across the British Isles, the high social visibility of orphans produced by famine conditions animated discussion in Ireland and sparked concern about the future moral development of Irish society. Post-Famine debates on child criminals were typically alarmist in nature, as evidenced by the inspectors-general's warnings of the 'great social peril' to arise from the 'corruption of the rising generation'. Their proposed solution involved shielding the destitute young institutionally from the demoralizing influences of adverse social conditions then thought to foster criminal tendencies. This step, the inspectors suggested, would ensure that the rising generation never became 'a moral pest and a burden on the public purse'. Instead, they were to be 'converted into orderly and self-supporting members of the community'.[2]

These perspectives can be neatly situated within a pervasive mid-nineteenth-century discourse on criminality that framed juvenile delinquency as an outcome of parental absence (due to being orphaned, abandoned or neglected) and a consequent lack of exposure to the moralizing influences of the domestic sphere.[3] Contemporary social thought privileged the home as a crucial site where, if in good order, children were appropriately socialized.[4] According to this precept, it was at home that children absorbed moral values of honesty and obedience. Contrarily, rearing in criminal settings inverted the normal processes believed to promote normative physical and moral growth. In England, the idea that children were being indoctrinated by criminals was immortalized in Charles Dickens' *Oliver Twist*, in which the master criminal Fagin trains children to pickpocket in his 'academy' in exchange for accommodation.[5]

The Famine coincided with mounting apprehension about the adverse physical and mental conditions caused by degrading social environments, and, more specifically, the ways in which poverty shaped morals, moulded criminal personalities and impacted detrimentally on bodily health. Mapping the so-called 'moral physiognomy' of London's outcast poor in the late 1840s, prominent journalist and social reformer Henry Mayhew had recently argued that physical, mental and moral degradation stemmed directly from hardship. Mayhew suggested that widespread poverty across Britain had created a social substratum referred to as the 'dangerous classes': a brutish sub-race or tribe-like group who tended not to be politically dangerous but who were worryingly prone to attacking properties and undertaking trivial, but socially disruptive, criminal acts.[6] Within Mayhew's framework, criminals were presented as both physically and mentally different from the more respectable classes and portrayed as a violent, savage race.[7] They appeared physically degenerate as they often suffered from conditions such as scrofula (or tuberculosis of the neck). Psychological deficiencies ensured that they possessed relatively limited moral control, while as a collective group they presented a worrying form of social pathology.[8] In essence, poverty and criminality took on indelible corporeal and psychological forms – acting as conditions that permeated, and became inscribed upon, the physical and mental makeup of criminals. Anxiety about the 'dangerous classes' in post-Famine Dublin can therefore be simultaneously interpreted as a response to the social cost of famine and as an assimilation of broader cultural attitudes to poverty that emphasized the emotive issue of juvenile criminality. These combined to promote a growing public awareness of the social condition of destitute, neglected and orphaned children.[9] Given the desire of the inspectors-general of prisons to 'convert' children into orderly, self-supporting beings, it is unsurprising that the institutional techniques imagined to tackle and regulate juvenile criminality focused intently upon reforming the bodies and minds of the destitute young.

This intersection of bodily concerns with post-Famine regimes of institutional child welfare has not been well documented. However, it is a crucial theme that requires consideration when analysing the development of Ireland's reformatory and industrial school system. Tom Feeney has persuasively argued that the idea of reforming criminal children was popularized in Ireland during the 1920s and 1930s when child guidance clinics became fashionable; sites where behaviour deemed deviant could be medically and psychologically rectified.[10] However, Feeney's arguments fail to recognize a longer genealogy of managing child deviance in Ireland that had much in common with early twentieth-century interventions. Although abandoned, neglected and orphaned children were assimilated into a range of institutions following the Famine – including orphanages, ragged schools and workhouses – mid-nineteenth-century reformatories and industrial schools served as key sites of bodily, psychological and moral reform.[11] In recent years the system, as a historical artefact, has been intensely criticized and scrutinized in response to internationally publicized allegations of sustained child abuse having surfaced.[12] Recent historical literature pertaining to these institutions tends to mirror modern perspectives by adopting an understandable, but somewhat biased, strategy of uncovering historical accounts of abuse and neglect.[13] Conor Reidy, for instance, places the phrase 'moral hospital' in inverted commas in the title of his recent study of early twentieth-century borstals – a narrative act presumably intended to suggest the irony of the words 'moral' and 'hospital' when applied to sites now commonly associated with sexual abuse and violence.[14]

Yet if we are to fully understand the historical development of Irish institutional provision for children, and, indeed, to appreciate what was actually meant by the label 'moral hospital', it is crucial to fully contextualize its origins and to avoid routinely imposing negative preconceptions on our historical conceptions of these institutions. Accordingly, within this chapter I probe into the bio-psychological paradigms that underpinned 'moral hospitals' and chart how childhood health was negotiated and managed with reference to a historically specific set of concerns over juvenile criminality. I begin by suggesting that criminality was understood within an organic framework that identified the bodies and minds of child criminals as having abnormally developed in the absence of nurturing parental influence. This precept played a formative role in the development of Irish reformatories and industrial schools, sites that emphasized the utility of both bodily and psychological reform as mechanisms that might re-establish normative patterns of physical, mental and moral growth. I continue by demonstrating that reformatories and industrial schools were initially designed as healthy environments juxtaposed to the criminal settings where the 'dangerous classes' were reared. Accordingly, institutional regimes targeted the physiological and psychological roots of criminality. As illustrative examples, I explore the multiple uses of outdoor work and diet as tools to reinstate normative growth. I conclude by suggesting that although these ideas remained predominant, other forms of medical superintendence evolved as new institutional health demands surfaced and as shifting forms of biological knowledge – in particular germ theory – required incorporation into institutional bodily strategies of governance. Importantly, the forms of illness and disease encountered in reality were often not those that medical thought had initially connected to criminality, meaning that these institutions ultimately came to, or were forced to, provide services bordering upon paediatric healthcare. Overall, I explore what reformatories and industrial schools were intended to be to further our knowledge of their development and to provide an alternative narrative that complements critical commentary on how these sites gradually transformed into places where the sanctity of childhood was threatened and undermined.

POVERTY, CRIME AND CHILDHOOD

In the mid-nineteenth century, numerous commentators perceived crime resulting from poverty as highly problematic for Ireland's social infrastructure and future national development. Despite being the second largest city in the British Isles, Dublin suffered from particularly acute, pervasive poverty while limited national industrialization ensured that rural Ireland continued to suffer from conditions of intense hardship for decades after the Famine.[15] Retrospectively analysing Ireland's criminal statistics during 1858, the *Dublin University Magazine* noted a peak in crimes against people and property during the Famine that had gradually declined from 1851. Yet despite these falling crime rates, the specific problem of juvenile crime had risen.[16] It is not clear whether incidence of juvenile criminality was genuinely increasing, or child criminals became more likely to be arrested due to their targeting as a social problem. Nonetheless, the issue maintained an undeniably high social visibility throughout the 1850s.

As noted above, Mayhewian thought dictated that the problem of 'outcast' children needed to be redressed if the social problem of criminality was to be resolved. These ideas were picked up on in Ireland. For instance, in a pamphlet on pauperism and national education published in 1857, Poor Law Union clerk John Taylor emotively portrayed Ireland as swarming with the 'dangerous classes' and urged the state to 'foster-father' the 'wretched little orphans that it leaves to be thrust into jail and ragged schools' so that these children could be elevated from a condition of 'savageism'.[17] Moral panic was also heightened by the existence of a sensationalized public discourse on child criminality.[18] The growth of a cheap Irish national and local press in the 1850s generated further public anxiety as audiences became exposed to hyperbolic statements published in newspapers including the *Irish Times*. On one occasion, that newspaper warned that youths released from prison were 'thoroughly impregnated with evil, and ten times more dangerous than before'.[19] Child crime was by no means a new phenomenon, but a distinct construct of juvenile delinquency was forged in this period and routinely applied in public discussion of the matter. The discourses that this enabled in Ireland allowed contemporaries to form responses to endemic poverty, overcrowded housing and widespread disease.[20] Concerned onlookers cited a range of causative factors directly tied to poverty, including inadequate housing arrangements, the absence of an appropriate system of industrial training in Ireland and low national wages. As the inspectors-general asserted in 1852, 'if these grave defects are found to operate injuriously in England, how much more severely must they be felt in Ireland, where the wretchedness and filth of the habitations of the poor almost furnish an apology for turning the children into the streets'.[21]

Importantly, official and medical perspectives framed juvenile delinquency within an organic framework that interpreted crime as a quasi-disease entity in itself. Its aetiological origins lay in the moral contagion generated by association with well-seasoned adult criminals. In this model, crime could be construed as a problem whose seeds were planted in early life, leaving enduring, possibly permanent, physical, psychological and moral imprints. These ideas were palpable in emerging ideas regarding the segregation of well-seasoned adult criminals and budding child criminals. During the 1850s, the inspectors-general pondered the best means of arresting 'the growth and full development of the dangerous classes within the very walls of institutions designed for their repression and correction' and proposed constructing separate institutions for youths. The additional expenditure that this would incur was justified with promises of the reduced financial burdens placed on future ratepayers. In the inspectors-general's phraseology, 'surely, if we follow the analogy of physical disease, this [the existing prison system] is to be found a costly hospital for advanced consumption'. Instead, future savings could be ensured by spending 'a small outlay and timely aid from the earlier symptoms of a comparatively trifling ailment'.[22] Evidently, child criminality came to be viewed practically and metaphorically as an illness requiring treatment.

A model was found in the influential ideas of educationalist and social reformer Mary Carpenter, whose concepts proved central to the development of the English reformatory school system and whose work was routinely referred to by the architects of the corresponding Irish system.[23] Carpenter had identified an impoverished class of young English children as 'perishing' due to an absence of appropriate parental influence. This 'perishing' class then became 'dangerous' by posing a distinct threat to social harmony with their criminal acts. For Carpenter, to be in a 'perishing' condition was to suffer from a 'grievous moral disease' requiring cure in what she termed a 'moral hospital'. There, physical and mental therapy would be 'guided by the highest wisdom of those who learnt the art of healing from the Physician of souls'.[24]

Carpenter detailed the work undertaken in 'moral hospitals' as analogous to that of a physician – a figure who, when investigating disease, carefully traced and noted symptoms, inquired into the habits and manners of his patients, ascertained whether illness was constitutional or occasioned by accident and then attempted to remove the deep seat of the malady before it worsened.[25] To further validate her pathologization of juvenile criminality, Carpenter identified children as physically and mentally immature, a social grouping whose muscles, bones and brains were in an incomplete state of growth. Conversely, however, the muscular and mental powers of 'perishing' children seemed to have prematurely developed as juvenile criminals took on overly active and independent roles deemed unsuited and unhealthy for their age. According to Carpenter's model, the will of juvenile criminals had acquired an unnatural strength unchecked by authority or reason, while forms of intellectual development had occurred that encouraged the gratification of animal desires rather than a spiritual nature.[26] By pathologizing juvenile criminality, Carpenter was well placed to develop a model of institutional reform that proved more attentive to the physical and psychological needs of the young, and which offered an alternative to the systems of stern, curative discipline found in prisons.[27]

Notably, reformatories and industrial schools were also conceived of in an era of shifting ideas on childhood and penal punishment. Early-Victorian approaches to prison management had emphasized punishment rather than personal reform. During the 1840s, the state had begun experimenting with modern penitentiaries, institutions where inmates were compelled to feel penitent about their sins through the imposition of harsh punishments including separate cells and enforced solitary confinement.[28] These disciplinary regimes seemed less suitable for youths. In fact, the suitability of prisons as sites of juvenile reform was widely questioned by the 1850s.[29] Margaret May has also suggested that the reformatory movement embodied a new conception of childhood as intrinsically different from adulthood, and which, accordingly, required differential attention.[30] May's perspectives are validated in nineteenth-century Irish contexts. For instance, Dublin barrister Patrick Joseph Murray, in his *Reformatories for Ireland* (1858), emotively argued that 'a child, even when criminal, should be treated as a child, and sent to a reformatory school and not a prison'. Foreseeing the improved social good that such a system would produce, Murray added that 'by the reformation of the young offender the country will be relieved from the cost of repeated convictions; from the expense of his prison support; from the evil of his corrupting example; and from the loss which his habits of plundering inflict on the community'.[31]

Similarly, when prominent social reformer and philanthropist James Haughton spoke to the Statistical Society of Dublin in 1857, he presented a persuasive case for curbing juvenile criminality through education as a means of elevating Ireland socially and morally.[32] Mark O'Shaughnessy, also speaking to the society, suggested that education might curb juvenile criminality and promote social and national improvement.[33] Evidently, debates on youth crime fused notions of individual, personal reform with broader strategies of social and national improvement. In these models, the bodies and minds of the young were inexorably linked to the well-being of Ireland as a whole.

Education was prioritized as it offered a way to restore positive moral and physical growth. An illuminating example of contemporary Irish thought on the matter can be found in physician and medical writer Thomas More Madden's *On Insanity and the Criminal Responsibility of the Insane* (1866) in which he depicted a young boy's descent into crime as follows:

> In this case we find a boy originally of a low order of intellect, of limited capacity, vain, frivolous, and of weak resolution, whose education and moral discipline evidently appear to have been neglected, and whose only reading was the lowest class of sensational literature, full of thrilling tales of crime and mystery. This kind of reading engaged his entire leisure, and evidently filled his imagination; so that like Don Quixote he surrounded himself with a world of fiction, which shaped his subsequent mania. Thus the autobiography, the attempted murder, and abortive suicide, all bear the impress of this mental dram-drinking.[34]

Madden portrayed the criminal boy as suffering from a form of 'moral insanity': an expression of mental disorder marked by 'hallucination of the morals' but without any obvious derangement of the intellectual powers. Crime itself became depicted as 'the result of an involuntary and irresistible mental malady by which all freedom of volition and of action are destroyed'.[35]

As part of this shifting tide in public opinion, reformatory schools were established in Ireland during 1858. The Industrial Schools (Ireland) Act of 1868 was predicated as an 'upgrade' for reformatories.[36] Reformatories were intended for children under the age of 16 who were guilty of offences while industrial schools provided for the neglected, orphaned or abandoned with high potential to become exposed to crime.[37] Each institution was independently managed, but subject to state approval and inspection.[38] Due to clerical demands for control and fears of proselytism, reformatory schools were run by different creeds and contained individuals of the same religion.[39]

Yet the underlying organic framework that underpinned contemporary conceptions of crime ensured that the bodies and minds of the institutionalized were routinely targeted for the purposes of reforming and improving.

BODILY AND PSYCHOLOGICAL REGIMES IN THE 'MORAL HOSPITAL'

If juvenile delinquency was so frequently understood in organic terms, what practical implications did this have for the day-to-day running of reformatories and industrial schools? The Industrial Feeding Schools, founded in Aberdeen in 1841, offered a suitable model as these had similarly implemented preventative, rather than punitive, systems. The experience of the Feeding Schools confirmed, to some, that the well-being of destitute youths improved when provided with food, training and religious instruction.[40] In 1868, John Lentaigne was appointed as inspector of Irish reformatories and, later, as inspector of industrial schools. Lentaigne was a prominent Dublin-born physician, and also the son of Dr Benjamin Lentaigne, a French royalist who had fled from Normandy to Dublin in 1792. John Lentaigne graduated with a medical degree in 1828, and later served in various administrative roles at Dublin Castle including Inspector-General of Prisons and Commissioner of Education.[41] He was instrumental in shaping Irish reformatories and industrial schools, which by 1884 housed 5,049 children nationwide. Given Lentaigne's robust medical background, it is unsurprising that the institutions under his inspection quickly came to serve quasi-medical purposes. Certainly, in his annual reports Lentaigne meticulously reported on the health and general management of individual reformatories and industrial schools, judging their working order with reference to the standards set by Carpenter's work. As Jane Barnes notes, Lentaigne exerted a remarkable influence in the early development of the system.[42]

In what ways, then, were reformatories and industrial schools constructed as healthy sites of reform and personal improvement? And in what ways did the medical world that surrounded Lentaigne shape how he practically managed those institutions? Ideally, institutional regimes directly targeted the physical, psychological and moral processes implicated as responsible for juvenile criminality. Lentaigne was initially sceptical of admitting children transferred from prisons whose health seemed particularly delicate. As he eloquently wrote, 'prisons and reformatories have been called moral hospitals; it is not, however, just or reasonable to convert them into physical ones'.[43] Elaborating, he expressed his view that reformatories could never provide a 'semi-miraculous cure' for crippling conditions such as scrofula, although they could, in some cases, alleviate their development.[44]

Nonetheless, Lentaigne's detailed reports of individual institutions indicate that many children who found their way there were in fact far from healthy. In one instance, he remarked that many children, upon arrival, were:

> … stunted in mind and in body, having the appearance of mere infants when in reality six or eight years of age, in nearly every case infected with disease – the offspring of poverty and neglect – poor and naked, with every loveliness of childhood banished from their countenance, and in some few, the germs of vice already deeply rooted.[45]

Lentaigne explicitly interpreted scrofula, as well as ophthalmia, consumption, epilepsy and forms of weak intellect, as symptomatic of imperfect nurturing in early life.[46] Accordingly, he intervened by attempting to restore natural nurturing influences in healthy environments. Importantly, Lentaigne's approaches shared commonalities with 'moral treatment'; a humane form of psychosocial care popularized throughout the nineteenth century and which, as Mark Finnane demonstrates in the Irish context, focused upon altering states of mind and producing socially tolerable behaviour. This was deemed achievable through education, religious training, agricultural work, the promotion of physical health, recreation and the redirecting of intellectual energies. Moral treatment had also emerged as a response to the harsh, physical regimes of punishment directed at the mentally ill throughout the eighteenth century.[47]

This multifaceted agenda was, for instance, clearly visible in Lentaigne's approach to the educational training of the criminal young. Unlike criminal environments, institutional education sought to render pupils self-reliant, laborious and capable of self-control, and to remove 'the feelings and ideas which surround abject poverty and crime'. This, in turn, was thought to equip destitute children with a psychological outlook required to obtain a better social positioning in later adult life.[48] Lentaigne, like Carpenter, believed that agricultural labour equipped students with a set of skills usefully transferable to later life. He simultaneously praised the healthy, invigorating influence of outdoor labour for its positive moral, mental and physical effects. Agricultural labour was portrayed as physically beneficial to child bodies; its variety was presented as mentally beneficial, while caring for animals was thought to awaken kind sympathies that would inspire the young to be more caring citizens.[49] The content of these educational regimes illuminates the ways in which the physicality and psychology of juvenile criminality was tackled on multiple levels and with reference to a wide, but interconnected, array of physical, psychological and moral regimes.

Importantly, outdoor labour also served disease management purposes. By emphasizing the physical benefits of agricultural labour, Lentaigne tapped into influential strands of medical thought that stressed the importance of fresh air in helping to prevent the development of conditions such as scrofula frequently encountered among destitute children. Prominent Irish surgeon Richard Carmichael and London-based surgeon Benjamin Philips were key medical authors on the disfiguring condition, and both had connected their observations of high urban incidence rates to the detrimental physical effects of unhealthy air. Their ideas underpinned curative principles for scrofula that viewed exposure to fresh countryside air positively. Earlier that century, Carmichael had depicted certain airs as possessing the ability to suppress processes of perspiration, meaning that vapours, rather than leaving the body, became trapped in the lungs which, in turn, affected the quality of digestive juices and ultimately predisposed individuals to scrofula.[50] By the time Philips published an influential medical text on the complaint in the 1840s, emphasis had shifted towards understanding towns and cities as producing unhealthy atmospheric environments that encouraged the onset of scrofula. By this period, medical emphasis was placed on issues of sanitation and public health. For instance, a key problem cited was a lack of ventilation in the dwellings of labourers believed to encourage contamination.[51] Nonetheless, fresh air persisted as an important mechanism of health restoration. On one occasion, Lentaigne wrote that 'the experience of my life satisfies me that scrofula and crime are intimately connected'.[52] Scrofula did indeed form the key target of institutional regimes, although open-air management was also occasionally recommended for other complaints. For example, following a number of cases of acute mania diagnosed among girls from High Park Reformatory for Roman Catholic Girls in Dublin, Lentaigne, in conjunction with an inspector of lunatic asylums, arranged for further outdoor employment to stifle the onset of further psychiatric illness.[53]

The example of agricultural work reveals the multiple levels on which individual elements of institutional life were intended to operate and the ways in which health, disease management and criminality became conceptually and practically linked. Agricultural labour equipped destitute children with transferable skills; strengthened bodies, minds and morals; generated desirable psychological mindsets; and, above all, ameliorated the pressing social concern of post-Famine juvenile criminality. In essence, agricultural labour offered a holistic regime of healthcare with observable individual and socio-national benefits. It also represented a Foucauldian-esque shift to subtle displays of bio-power and bio-politics that sought to govern and reshape institutionalized subjects through the regulation of the body.[54]

Diet also proved central to Lentaigne's vision of how to curb juvenile criminality. Poor infant and child feeding was routinely implicated as partly to blame for abnormal physical and mental growth. Good feeding, conversely, was understood as being imbued with the potential to halt the development of chronic illness, restore normative processes of childhood growth, and fulfil the overarching goal of achieving bodily, psychological and moral salvation. For Lentaigne, if children were underfed when young, tendencies to pursue an immoral lifestyle increased. More specifically, Lentaigne explicitly drew from the writings of German internist physician Felix Von Niemeyer, who had achieved fame for pioneering a high-protein, low carbohydrate diet. Niemeyer identified coarse diets containing little nutriment as a prime cause of scrofula. In his model, the tender organs of infants had failed to assimilate appropriate levels of nutriment at an early age, rendering them liable to the disease. The outcome, for Niemeyer, was impoverished and vitiated circulation and children growing with impaired nervous powers, devoid of energy or vigour and deficient in self-control and self-reliance.[55] Conversely, good feeding encouraged the normal development of muscular, cerebral and mental functions, and prevented the onset of diseases understood as resulting from low vitality and weak blood.[56]

Medicinal foods such as cod liver oil were also given to scrofulous children. For instance, Lentaigne reported that at Moate Industrial School, County Westmeath, 'some [children] have drunk more than their weight of that valuable medicine since their admission', while large quantities of eggs were supplied to suffering children at St Martha's Industrial School, County Monaghan.[57] Yet the organic framework underpinning contemporary perceptions of the aetiology of scrofula also, and sometimes controversially, legitimated healthy, varied and generous food provisions.[58] In his annual reports, Lentaigne regularly lambasted institutional managers who fed destitute children with inadequate combinations of bread, milk, stirabout and Indian meal; promoting generous feeding instead.[59] He did face occasional public criticism for recommending provisions significantly higher than those offered in workhouses and prisons.[60] Yet, in response, he argued that, unlike workhouses, industrial schools were not intended to rescue people from starvation but instead to act in *loco parentis* to children and to prepare them for a healthy physical, moral and social existence.[61] Reformatories and industrial schools were therefore intended to serve as sites that were attentive to health in ways that workhouses and prisons tended not to be to the same degree.[62] Broadly holistic models of health were applied that posited close connections between physical health, mental processes and

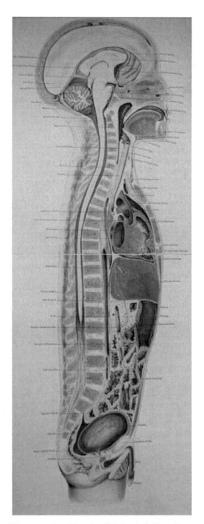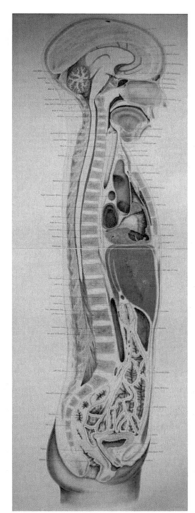

Figure 1. Vertical Mesial Section of Body of Boy aged Six Years' and 'Vertical Mesial Section of Body of Girl aged Thirteen Years', in J. Symington, *The Topographical Anatomy of the Child* (London: Bailliere, Tindall & Cox, 1887), Plates I and II, pp.9, 11.

Reproduced by kind permission of the Royal College of Physicians of Ireland.

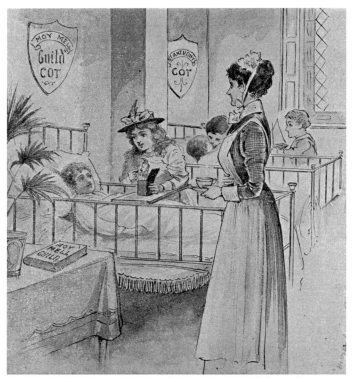

Figure 2. Line Drawing of the Moy Mell Children's Guild, Temple Street, in *Twenty-Eighth Annual Report of the Children's Hospital Temple Street and Report of the Moy Mell Children's Guild* (Dublin, 1901).
Courtesy of Temple Street Children's University Hospital.

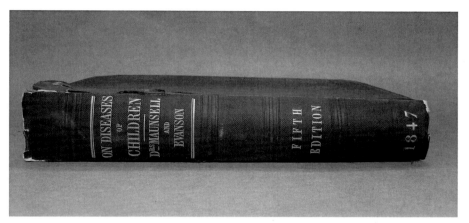

Figure 3. Photograph of R.T. Evanson and H. Maunsell, *A Practical Treatise on the Management and Diseases of Children,* 3rd edn (Dublin: Fannin, 1840). Reproduced by kind permission of the Royal College of Physicians of Ireland.

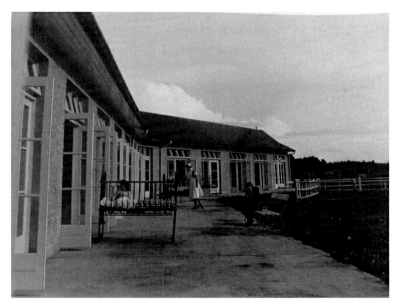

Figure 4. Undated photograph of the Children's Sunshine Home, Stillorgan (Overend Archive, Airfield Trust, Dublin). Reproduced by kind permission of Kathy Purcell, Director, Airfield Trust.

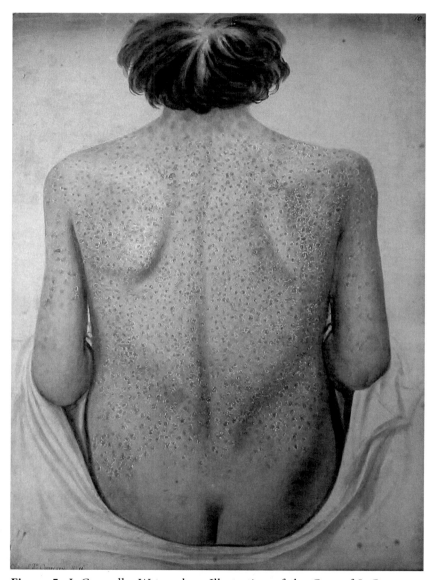

Figure 5. J. Connolly, Watercolour Illustration of the Case of J. Courtney, aged 11. Illustration shows Courtney's back which is covered in a rash caused by syphilis in the mid-nineteenth century (Royal College of Physicians of Ireland, MI/1/9).

Reproduced by kind permission of the Royal College of Physicians of Ireland.

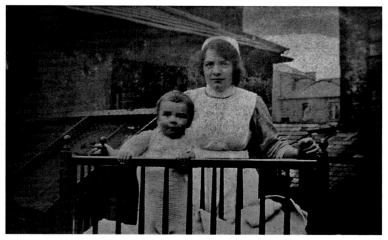

Figure 6. Kevin – 13 months at St Ultan's Hospital, 23 April 1923 (Royal College of Physicians of Ireland, St Ultan's Hospital photographic album 1919-29, (SU/8/3/1).
Reproduced by kind permission of the Royal College of Physicians of Ireland.

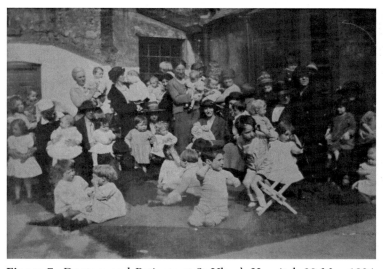

Figure 7. Doctors and Patients at St Ultan's Hospital, 30 May 1924 (Royal College of Physicians of Ireland, St Ultan's Hospital photograph album 1919–29, SU/8/3/1).
Reproduced by kind permission of the Royal College of Physicians of Ireland.

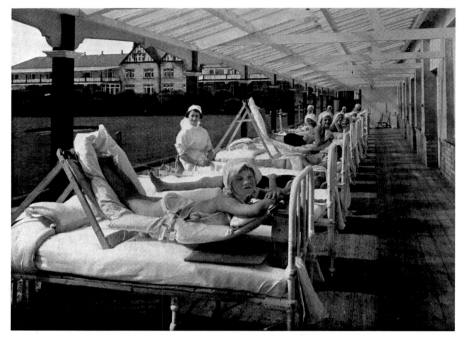

Figure 8. 'Senior Girls – Surgical Cases': Patients at Stannington Sanatorium, Morpeth, Northumberland, the first British sanatorium for tuberculosis illustrating immobilisation techniques for tuberculous children.
Reproduced by kind permission of the Wellcome Library, London.

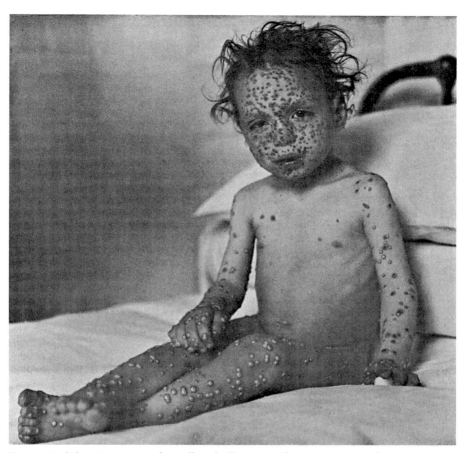

Figure 9. 'The Diagnosis of Smallpox': illustrates the appearance of smallpox in a small child (T.F. Ricketts, Casell & Company, 1908).
Reproduced by kind permission of the Wellcome Library, London.

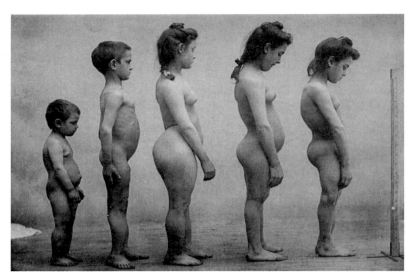

Figure 10. 'Male and Female Children with Rickets – Side View, c. 1901', in Masson and Cie (eds), *Nouvelle Iconographie de la Salpétrière; Clinique des Maladies du Système Nerveus* (Paris: Libraires de l'Academie de Medecine, c. 1901), Tome XIV, Plate XLIV.
Reproduced by kind permission of the Wellcome Library, London.

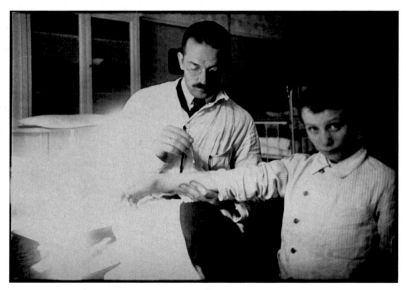

Figure 11. Clemens von Pirquet and a patient.
Reproduced by kind permission of the Wellcome Library, London.

moral behaviour. In doing so, steps were taken to ensure a normal growth into adulthood that, in turn, allowed reformatories and industrial schools to develop into institutions that emphasized the preservation of child health through regimes of labour and diet.

MANAGING CHILDHOOD ILLNESS

Lentaigne once asserted that moral hospitals were never intended as physical hospitals, as cited above. But to what extent was this agenda sustainable? Moral hospitals might well have been designed principally as preventative sites. Yet, as they evolved, managers were obliged to manage and cure bodily complaints not always obviously connected to the physicality of criminality. This raises a pertinent question: did the work of institutional managers coalesce entirely around acting as moral guardians or did it also entail other forms of medical superintendence? Certainly, as medical knowledge evolved throughout the late nineteenth century, Irish reformatories and industrial schools metamorphosed into sites where nascent forms of biomedical knowledge needed to be applied in institutional healthcare regimes. Although initially configured to promote bodily, psychological and moral improvement, the need to manage and contain disease ensured that reformatories and industrial schools ultimately, and mostly accidentally, came to provide quasi-paediatric services. Throughout the late nineteenth century, these sites began focusing just as much on cure as prevention, while the nature of diseases requiring management gradually expanded beyond the physical conditions such as scrofula that had, in the 1850s, been linked to criminality. Importantly, Lentaigne's capacity as both physician and government inspector equipped him with an up-to-date awareness of the rapidly shifting forms of late nineteenth-century medical knowledge which, in turn, enabled him to direct effective regimes of institutional health management in Ireland.

Notably, deaths from epidemic diseases in these institutions were remarkably low, especially in comparison to workhouses, which were perennially criticized for high rates of mortality among the young.[63]

During 1870, only seven deaths in industrial schools were recorded from a national average population of 1,289 inmates, or 0.54 per cent of inmates.[64] By contrast, workhouse mortality per week in the same year was as high (nationally) as 4.1 per cent.[65] Importantly, Lentaigne actively encouraged managers to familiarize themselves with the most current strands of medical thought and to apply these when caring for institutionalized children. For instance, responding to observations of high incidence rates of institutional ophthalmia (or inflammation of the eye), Lentaigne drew attention to the research of prominent British physician and ophthalmic surgeon Robert Brudenall Carter who, in his influential *Diseases of the Eye* (1876), depicted widespread ophthalmic complaints among 'street Arabs' and orphans as a consequence of insufficient feeding in early life. Lentaigne used these ideas to further validate generous food provisions, especially for those suffering from the condition.[66] Some institutions even evolved into specialist sites where problems of childhood blindness were managed. From the 1870s, for example, blind girls were sent from local workhouses to Merrion Industrial School for Roman Catholic Girls, County Dublin where visually able girls were trained to nurse and administer to the needs of the blind.[67]

Importantly, however, this marked emphasis on physical and psychological reform was complemented by new, increasingly necessary, medical techniques once germ theory gradually became accepted. In this context, dietary and environmental management *alone* appeared as less suitable techniques for checking disease as epidemiological, rather than environmental and constitutional, configurations became gradually accepted as aetiologically important.[68] For instance, in 1880 when scarlatina broke out in St Nicholas' Industrial School, Cork, resident boys were provided with meat each day for curative purposes. Yet, suspecting that germs might be the aetiological origin of the disease, Lentaigne informed managers that controlling the disease dietetically was impossible when 'the spores of contagion are floating through the atmosphere in a disease-stricken district'.[69]

Acting reactively to rapid biomedical discoveries, throughout the 1880s Lentaigne implemented important changes in institutional management. For example, he urged managers to isolate the sick in separate infirmaries or rooms and to disinfect personal belongings, vociferously lambasting those who failed to do so. These adjustments were predicated on the basis that 'particles, which are generally believed to be living organisms, may be carried in the dust by the winds, or in the sewer gas from the drains, and when once admitted into the system they propagate and multiply'.[70] Lentaigne also promoted structural changes, including the removal of lavatories from bedrooms. This idea stemmed from notions that ophthalmic germs spread rapidly among children sleeping in environments where cleanliness was not properly observed.[71] Similarly, in 1882 Lentaigne cited Irish physicist John Tyndall's announcement in *The Times* of German bacteriologist Robert Koch's famed discovery of the bacterial origin of tuberculosis and immediately urged managers to isolate tuberculosis victims to prevent transmission through air.[72] Evidently, Lentaigne was instrumental in promoting health regimes not explicitly connected to the onset of criminal tendencies in models such as Carpenter's or in the psychosocial writings of Madden. Although an insistence on healthy environments persisted, how those environments were managed adjusted swiftly as biomedical thought shifted.

As well as being well versed in bacteriological theory, Lentaigne was also attuned to the need to inspect child health, a step being slowly initiated in institutions and schools more generally.[73] Although these schemes were implemented at a far slower pace in Ireland in comparison to England, Lentaigne sponsored their introduction early on. By the late 1880s he sought to tackle conditions including ophthalmia through frequent medical inspections, close attention to lavatory arrangements, and the isolation of acute cases. Ringworm (a fungal disease of the skin) also became managed through the provision of separate towels, combs and brushes, coupled with regular medical inspection.[74] Incidentally, by 1890 Lentaigne's son, also named John, was reported to be treating scrofula using the latest surgical techniques.[75]

Evidently, the means of institutionally tackling the perceived physical and psychological roots of juvenile criminality were considered in multiple ways within the Irish reformatory and industrial school system. Disease prevention had always been crucial to the discourses surrounding the institutionalization of the young. In particular, physical diseases such as scrofula had been directly linked to the physicality of the 'dangerous classes'. Yet an ideological framework that prioritized tackling disease in its early stages was ultimately complemented, if not supplanted, by a broader range of medical techniques. This facilitated the development of a more fluid, adaptable system of healthcare.

CONCLUSIONS

Criminality was broadly construed as a physical, psychological and moral problem in post-Famine Ireland. As child criminality became linked to abnormal bodily and mental growth, new techniques of governing bodies, minds and morals surfaced and became embodied in the preventative and curative agendas of reformatories and industrial schools. In turn, enormous social benefits were promised due to the diminished threat posed by the 'dangerous classes' – a group whose population threatened to perpetually increase following the Famine, a catastrophe that had dislocated many children from the natural, nurturing influence of the domestic sphere. The institutional contexts in which child health now had to be negotiated and managed fostered a system that aspired to provide forms of paediatric care. Understanding the historical interplay between institutional power and the bodies of the young will prove to be a central concern of social historians of Ireland in future years in light of ongoing revelations of sexual scandals. In this chapter, I have considered one, perhaps more positive, avenue where this power was displayed: through the creation of institutionalized bio-populations subject to techniques of physical, psychological and moral reform. Exploring the ideological roots of Irish institutional childcare illuminates what that system was initially meant to be and therefore serves as a useful reference point for understanding how it ultimately transmuted into a more controversial space of childhood.

7

The Penny Test: Tuberculin Testing and Paediatric Practice in Ireland, 1900–1960

Anne Mac Lellan

 y means of the skin test, which takes one minute and costs one penny, primary infection can be recognized at its inception.[1]

Dorothy Price

Mortality from tuberculosis was in decline by the mid-nineteenth century in most European countries. However, the Irish epidemic peaked in 1904.[2] After this date, the number of deaths from tuberculosis in Ireland went into a gradual decline, with interruptions during the two world wars when mortality due to tuberculosis temporarily rose.[3] The rate of decline was slow, and the proportionate fall in mortality due to tuberculosis in Ireland did not keep pace with other developed countries.[4] From 1927 to 1937, Ireland had the lowest annual percentage reduction in tuberculosis mortality among twenty countries in Europe, North America and Australasia.[5] There is no simple singular reason for Ireland's different experience of tuberculosis. In an international context, the role of social and economic factors in the decline of epidemic tuberculosis has been increasingly foregrounded since Thomas McKeown, in 1976, challenged the role of medicine in the decline of tuberculosis prior to 1935.[6] Arguments continue about the weighting that should be applied to factors such as decreasing virulence of the bacterium, increased host immunity, better housing, better nutrition, better-quality milk, improved public health measures, hospital bed provision, X-rays and antibiotics in addition to preventive interventions such as isolation and vaccination.[7] Greta Jones' detailed analysis of the trajectory of Ireland's tuberculosis epidemic in the nineteenth and twentieth centuries demonstrates the complex interplay of the variables that determined the course of the Irish epidemic. These included economic development and urbanization, overcrowding in urban settings, political considerations, emigration, poverty, nutrition, infected milk, public health and iatrogenic interventions.[8]

Tuberculosis is often presumed to be a chronic pulmonary disease affecting the lungs of adults, but the disease also affected children, with non-pulmonary forms of the disease outnumbering the pulmonary form in the first half of the twentieth century.[9] Tuberculosis could infect any part of a child's body including bones and joints, the abdomen and the membranes surrounding the brain as well as being disseminated throughout the body in millet-seed-sized nodules in a form of the disease known as 'miliary' tuberculosis.[10] In 1922, the year the independent Irish state was founded, a total of 4,614 deaths from tuberculosis were recorded in the country, 611 of which were among children under 15 years of age. By 1930, this had fallen to 537 (total deaths 3,825). Two decades later, in 1950, the death rate among children under the age of 15 fell to 232 deaths (total deaths 2,380). However, for much of the first half of the twentieth century, tuberculosis was the third leading cause of death among Irish children, eclipsed only by gastroenteritis and pneumonia.[11] Tuberculosis was more prevalent among children in urban settings, probably as a consequence of overcrowding in slum settings in cities such as Dublin.[12] The mortality figures for children in Dublin far exceeded those in comparable cities such as Manchester, Leeds and Copenhagen.[13] It was estimated that for every death, seven to nine people were ill with tuberculosis, so childhood tuberculosis presented a substantial challenge to the Irish medical profession as well as a threat to children's quality of life. As

Susan Kelly has discussed in this volume, Irish children with bone and joint tuberculosis had to endure long and painful illness even after antibiotics became available as these drugs had limited penetration into some body sites.

The official mortality figures for childhood deaths from tuberculosis in Ireland were probably an underestimate as misdiagnosis was common and death certificates were unreliable.[14] The Professor of Medicine in Trinity College Dublin, Victor Millington Synge, wrote that medical students walking the wards of Dublin's hospital in the 1920s were confronted with:

> … cases of tuberculous glands in the neck, tuberculosis of bones and joints, and tuberculous peritonitis, many of which recovered after a long illness. He [the medical student] also saw numerous cases of tuberculous meningitis and miliary tuberculosis. Nothing could be done for such cases – the victim always died in a few weeks. How a child acquired tuberculous meningitis or miliary tuberculosis was obscure. Tuberculin reactions were brushed aside as unreliable if not misleading.[15]

Tuberculin testing, mentioned by Synge in his retrospective analysis of the situation in the 1920s, is based on the fact that the introduction of tuberculin into a person who had been previously exposed to tuberculosis leads to a response, great or small, depending on the route of exposure and the dosage.[16] Children who tested negative to tuberculin had not been exposed to tuberculosis; they did not have any immunity against tuberculosis and were vulnerable to infection by the disease. These tuberculin-negative children came to be regarded as suitable subjects for preventive vaccination that would boost their immunity. A safe version of the tuberculin test had been developed in 1907, providing a reliable indication of infection with tuberculosis. Matters with respect to diagnosis of tuberculosis in Ireland did not improve substantially. Morgan Crowe, deputy chief medical officer, Dublin city, described the investigation of a suspected tubercular person prior to the 1940s as a 'rather haphazard affair' consisting largely of 'stethoscopic examination'. 'X-rays, tuberculin tests etc. were not in vogue here,' he wrote, and 'peculiarly enough, sputum testing seems to have been neglected'.[17]

As pointed out by Susan Kelly in this volume, the historiography of tuberculosis in Ireland has paid considerably more attention to the adult experience of the disease than to childhood forms of tuberculosis.[18] So it is not surprising that the use or neglect of tuberculin testing for diagnosis of tuberculosis in Irish children has been afforded little attention by historians.[19] This chapter will argue that the role of tuberculin testing in mitigating and mapping tuberculosis in Ireland between 1930 and 1960 is worthy of detailed attention in light of its usefulness both for diagnosis of tuberculosis infection in individual children and for epidemiological purposes. Children who were incorrectly diagnosed as tubercular might be prescribed long unnecessary periods of bed rest. They might also be placed in contact with active cases of tuberculosis if they were sent to a sanatorium for treatment. Conversely, children with undiagnosed tuberculosis might be deprived of the rest and treatment that they required.[20] At community level, a failure to trace contacts of the tubercular could allow for the unchecked development of micro-epidemics in institutions, families and housing clusters. At national level, the lack of tuberculin testing added to the unreliability of regional and national statistics in respect of tuberculosis mortality and morbidity among both children and adults.

In addition to diagnosis of tuberculosis infection in individuals, tuberculin testing provided the means to map patterns of tuberculosis infection within various populations. As Anne Hardy has pointed out, in the British context the perception of tuberculosis altered between 1940 and 1970 following the publication of large-scale epidemiological studies that used tuberculin testing and X-rays to trace and diagnose tubercular illness. According to Hardy, the new techniques replaced the old 'romanticized image' of tuberculosis with one 'centred on children and the old'.[21] Epidemiological studies using tuberculin testing in Ireland were carried out in paediatric populations from the 1930s onwards. This chapter will extend Hardy's thesis to Ireland and point to the usefulness of Irish studies in altering the perception of Irish children's experience of tuberculosis. Finally, it will consider the impact of the development of strategies for the identification of cohorts of children at risk of contracting tuberculosis and the introduction of preventive strategies such as vaccination.

TUBERCULIN SKIN TESTS: DEVELOPMENT AND EARLY INDIFFERENCE

Tuberculin was first produced by the Prussian bacteriologist Robert Koch who, in 1882, had demonstrated that tuberculosis was caused by a bacterium. He quickly followed this up by controversially informing the medical world that he had manufactured a cure for tuberculosis called tuberculin.[22] In addition to proclaiming the curative properties of his 'secret foreign fluid', Koch recognized that it could be used as a diagnostic aid.[23] The fluid proved ineffective as a cure and was soon revealed to be nothing more complex than an extract of tubercular protein, produced by autoclaving, filtering and concentrating a culture of *Mycobacterium tuberculosis*.[24] Patients undergoing treatment began to get ill or die, while Koch was unable or unwilling to demonstrate the guinea pigs he had purportedly cured with it. In the wake of much adverse publicity, many physicians abandoned the use of tuberculin in treatment.[25] A minority continued to proclaim its virtues as a cure for tuberculosis and injected their patients with preparations of varying potency for the next forty years.[26]

Meanwhile, early diagnostic tuberculin tests were unwieldy to perform and involved generalized whole-body reactions such as a rise in temperature. There were technical difficulties in standardizing tuberculin, problems with administration and methods of measuring the body's response. Then in 1907 a tuberculin skin test was devised in Vienna by the Austrian paediatrician and allergist Clemens von Pirquet.[27] Other skin tests were quickly developed, ranging from the more sensitive Mantoux, which required injection, to less sensitive ointments, jellies and patches that were applied to the intact skin and less painful to use and, hence, deemed more suitable for children.[28] If negative, these latter tests had to be repeated with more sensitive tests, but for children who tested positive with the initial test, no further tests were necessary. The importance of the skin test was that the reaction was local, making the test safer than the earlier tests. Tuberculin testing provided evidence of infection with tuberculosis, while X-rays were generally used to provide evidence of active infection. The continental medical profession began to incorporate tuberculin skin tests into its diagnostic algorithms.[29]

The Irish and British medical professions were slow to engage with diagnostic tuberculin testing, even in paediatric populations where researchers were agreed it had greatest value as children were less likely to have been exposed to tuberculosis and more likely to be tuberculin negative. Twenty years after methods of diagnosis were well established on the continent, the Irish paediatrician Dorothy Price ascribed the lack of engagement with diagnostic tuberculin testing in Ireland to the fact that doctors in Ireland did not read or visit German-speaking centres and 'took everything via England'.[30] However, while this may have been the case for the majority of doctors, there were exceptions such as the Dublin bacteriologist Edmond Joseph McWeeney who studied in Berlin and Vienna.[31] Moreover, there were some voices in favour of tuberculin testing in the British medical literature, although Francis Barrymore Smith has pointed out that Great Britain's principal proponents of tuberculin, Robert Philip in Edinburgh and W. Camac Wilkinson in London, were, ironically, also its worst enemies as they continued, up until the late 1920s, to discuss the two very different uses of tuberculin – as therapeutic agent and as diagnostic agent – in tandem, creating confusion about the place of tuberculin in tuberculosis.[32] In 1931, John Gibbens of St Thomas's Hospital, London highlighted the fact that the diagnostic tuberculin test was 'extensively used in all children's hospitals on the continent and in the USA, yet its usage in this country [Great Britain] is quite exceptional'.[33] In a suggestion that chimed with the continued development of paediatrics as a separate medical specialism in Great Britain, he suggested that the teaching of childhood tuberculosis should be taken out of the hands of the specialists in adult disease.[34] In 1933, Leonard Findlay, a physician in Princess Elizabeth of York Hospital for Children, London, suggested that the tuberculin test might have a role in diagnosing children under the age of 2.[35]

In Ireland, at least two small trials were carried out prior to 1910 in an attempt to assess the usefulness of tuberculin tests developed on the continent in the diagnosis of tuberculosis; one of these involved children.[36] This latter trial was carried out by the pathologist and bacteriologist McWeeney. Working in the Mater Misericordiae Hospital, Dublin, McWeeney compared von Pirquet's new skin test with an older methodology whereby tuberculin was introduced to the eye. Using a dilute solution of Koch's Old Tuberculin for the eye tests and a much stronger solution for the skin tests, he found the conjunctival test more useful. However, the 'unpleasantly vigorous reaction' in a few children with 'early tuberculous glands' meant that he reduced the strength by half, and now used 1 per cent tuberculin for the eye testing. Although McWeeney continued to use the eye as the site of introduction for tuberculin, its use was soon discredited as it could cause dangerous reactions.[37] There are no further reports of tuberculin testing trials involving the skin test in the Irish medical literature until the mid-1930s. In addition to being neglected by researchers, there is no evidence that tuberculin testing was used routinely by public health doctors, general practitioners or paediatricians in Ireland. This may have been partly due to the influence of the British medical profession, as posited by Price. It may also have been part of a general falloff in tackling infectious diseases as violent political upheaval enveloped Ireland from 1916 to 1923.[38] The very practice of reporting outbreaks of infectious diseases fell 'into disuse' in many districts.[39] The first report of the new Department of Local Government and Public Health, which dealt with the years from the foundation of the new Irish state in 1922 until 1925, noted that a 'gradual recovery' in public health services was being achieved.

CONTINENTAL INFLUENCES ON THE IRISH USE OF TUBERCULIN TESTING IN THE 1930s

A network of connections between Irish paediatricians and their colleagues in the medical profession on the continent was primarily responsible for the introduction of the tuberculin skin test into paediatric practice in Ireland. In 1931, Price visited the Kinderklinik in the Allgemeines Krankenhaus, Vienna. This visit, followed by her later observation of two cases of primary tuberculosis in twins, influenced Price to engage with tuberculin for diagnosis and to carry out a series of studies that were instrumental in its acceptance in Ireland.[40] The Kinderklinik was a world-renowned centre of paediatric medicine in Europe, combining research with clinical work and offering postgraduate courses.[41] Although Price was not primarily interested in tuberculosis at this time, she elected to follow the famous Professor Franz Hamburger on his rounds.[42] Impressed with his use of tuberculin skin testing, she brought back a tube of Hamburger's (tuberculin) ointment. In addition, she purchased various textbooks in German for which she procured the assistance of a translator before, very quickly, learning to read and speak the language herself, as she considered German medical literature on tuberculosis essential.[43]

Price, who worked as a physician in St Ultan's Hospital, Dublin, did not use the Hamburger's ointment that she had procured in Vienna until 1933 when she and her colleague Nora O'Leary tuberculin tested two sick twins in the hospital.[44] One twin, Peter, had a high temperature but did not appear to be very ill. At the suggestion of a doctor in the laboratory in Trinity College Dublin, Price did a tuberculin test using the Hamburger's ointment. The test was strongly positive. Louis, the other twin, was tuberculin negative but he soon developed a fever and his tuberculin test became positive. These two cases of primary tuberculosis were the 'first and also the most outstanding examples of initial fever' that Price encountered.[45] Thus, it was the concatenation of two chance events – following Hamburger on a ward round and, two years later, seeing twin boys develop primary tuberculosis – that interested Price in tuberculin testing. The boys, accompanied by O'Leary, went to a sanatorium in Scheidegg in Germany. Price later enrolled on a ten-day postgraduate course in Scheidegg. Studying alongside Danish, Swiss and German colleagues, and using her newly acquired German language skills, Price became even more convinced of the validity of continental views on tuberculosis, particularly with respect to diagnosis.[46] In her view, tuberculin testing, followed by X-ray, provided valuable evidence of infection. Price and O'Leary began to use the Hamburger's ointment on 'all and sundry', testing 100 inpatient babies in St Ultan's Hospital for infants and later extending the work to 246 outpatients in St Ultan's and the Royal City of Dublin Hospital. Price believed that early diagnosis, facilitated by tuberculin testing, was essential for the effective treatment of childhood tuberculosis.[47] Many children who were infected with tuberculosis recovered completely and were symptomless throughout their primary infection; however, in others the disease progressed, and rest was considered essential for recovery.[48] Children could only be healed of tuberculosis if they were diagnosed in the early or primary stage of the disease, according to Price. For her, the two crucial elements of treatment were the removal of infants from 'all possible tuberculous contact' and bed rest, both of which could be achieved by admission to hospital or a sanatorium, although there was a shortage of such beds.

As in Britain, the interest in the diagnosis and treatment of tuberculosis in children in Ireland paralleled and contributed to the development of paediatric medicine as a specialism. The Irish Paediatric Club, which later became the Irish Paediatric Association, was set up in 1933 by Robert Collis and its first meeting was held in Dorothy Price's home.[49] Writing in 1967, John Mowbray, a paediatrician at the Children's Hospital, Temple Street, Dublin, asserted that this club, with its 'pitifully small but indomitable membership', was responsible for the paediatrician 'being recognized as the equal of the consultant physician, surgeon and obstetrician'. Price and Collis shared a strong interest in the diagnosis and treatment of childhood tuberculosis. In 1934, Price and a colleague tuberculin tested the patients in the children's pavilion in Peamount Sanatorium, Dublin.[50] Fourteen out of 53 children reacted negatively. Dr Alice Barry, the Peamount superintendent, gradually sent these children home with a note to their County Medical Officer of Health (CMOH) explaining that they were not tubercular. Neither tuberculosis officers (TOs) nor CMOHs, who would have referred the children to the sanatorium, routinely used tuberculin tests at this time. All subsequent entries to Peamount children's pavilion were tuberculin tested on entry and the negatives were not admitted. However, there was no onus on other sanatoria to follow suit. Admission policies were developed at an institutional level rather than on a national basis, so children who may not have had tuberculosis continued to be admitted to institutions where they were immediately placed in contact with infectious cases of the disease.

The situation was very different in Scandinavian countries. In Sweden, in the early 1920s, the Swedish paediatrician Professor Arvid Wallgren had commenced his influential work with tuberculin testing and the preventive BCG vaccine in Gothenburg.[51] By the 1930s tuberculin skin tests were in universal use in Scandinavian schools, hospitals and other institutions. Collis visited Sweden in 1932 and brought Wallgren's work to Price's attention.[52] Price visited hospitals and laboratories in Norway, Sweden and Denmark in 1936 and 1938 and became an ardent emulator of Scandinavian medical practice with respect to childhood tuberculosis. The Scandinavian approach to tackling tuberculosis concentrated on 'disease-causing microbes' rather than 'disease-causing unhealthy habits'.[53] By 1938, Price had accrued five years' experience with diagnosing and treating infants with tuberculosis. Writing in the *British Medical Journal* in 1938, she expressed her belief in the need for early diagnosis; she highlighted the usefulness of tuberculin testing in achieving this diagnosis and suggested a regime of care for infants. The response to this article illustrates some of the difficulties facing practitioners, at community level, with respect to tuberculin testing.[54] The CMOH in Wicklow, Dr G.P.G. Beckett, wrote that she was correct that it was 'impossible to diagnose pulmonary TB in an infant by means of a stethoscope and extremely difficult in older children'.[55] Of the means of diagnosis – tuberculin skin test, radiography and history of contact – Beckett said that only the latter was 'practicable' as he had to attend twelve to fourteen TB dispensaries a month and had only a nurse in attendance for about half of those. It would be impossible for him to recall patients to read skin reactions and there was no 'efficient X-ray apparatus' in the county. There was a lack of information and no formal training available. The tuberculosis inspector at the Department of Local Government and Public Health, E.J.T. McWeeney (the son of Professor Edmond Joseph McWeeney), noted 'stigma and ignorance of early symptoms'. It was difficult to persuade parents to bring 'apparently healthy children', who had been in contact with tuberculosis, for examination. Education would combat this 'ignorance and misapprehension', according to E.J.T. McWeeney.[56]

In 1939, Price and Collis invited Wallgren to visit Dublin and he gave a lecture at the Royal College of Physicians of Ireland. Price used the visit to generate publicity about the value of the tuberculin test, which took only 'one minute and costs one penny'.[57] Wallgren told the meeting that in the city of Gothenburg the families of children who tested positive for tuberculosis were tuberculin tested and, in this way, new sources of infection were identified.[58] This lecture appeared to galvanize Irish TOs into using tuberculin testing. Prior to Wallgren's visit, only one Irish TO was using tuberculin. E.J.T. McWeeney optimistically told Price that all of the TOs were now using the tuberculin test on contact children.[59] However, Price continued to receive information from those working on the ground indicating that tuberculin was not easy to fit into the routine of a rural dispensary.[60]

TUBERCULIN TESTING IRISH CHILDREN IN THE 1940s

At national level, prior to the Second World War, the official engagement with tuberculin testing by the Department of Public Health and Local Government amounted to little more than the bestowal of approving notices on work being done on an *ad-hoc* basis. With the advent of the Second World War, pragmatic difficulties compounded official inertia, making it even more difficult for those doctors who wished to continue to tuberculin test children as Hamburger's ointment became unavailable. In 1943, Price made up a substitute ointment which she called Dublin Moro. It consisted of two parts Old Tuberculin and one part wool fat. Price gave it free of charge to those who asked her for it, mainly assistant CMOHs and doctors dealing with children.[61] The demand was such that she began to charge the cost price of the materials. Cost price worked out at less than one penny per test, provided the material was kept in a syringe and there was no waste. The Dublin Moro ointment was later made up by the National Vaccine Institute, Dublin.

The importance of continuing to use diagnostic tuberculin tests was underlined by Price in the 1940s, when she wrote that the death rate had been reduced among forty-eight infants under 2 years of age to 22 per cent compared with a previous death rate of almost 80 per cent in the 1930s.[62] She attributed the reduction in mortality to the use of routine tuberculin testing of all infants in the outpatients department of St Ultan's and by admission of these early cases, as well as more advanced cases, to a 'special fresh-air tuberculosis ward'. She emphasised that among infants under 3 months, the prognosis was 'extremely bad' no matter how early the diagnosis. In addition to removal from the source of infection, the enforcement of rest and the use of fresh air as a therapy, children in St Ultan's benefited from improved nutrition. Price's results bolster the suggestion by Anne Hardy that there is some evidence that 'care' did play a role, albeit undefined, in the survival of the tubercular individual.[63] The reduction in the death rate achieved by Price also speaks to Michael Worboys' discussion of 'significant innovations' in management and therapies, as doctors attempted to 'attack the seeds of disease' and, more importantly, the boosting of 'the condition of the human soil' so it could better resist the tubercle bacillus.[64]

Despite the wider use of the tuberculin test on Irish children, as evinced by the demand for Dublin Moro ointment, Collis upset his colleagues by alleging, in 1945, that half of the tubercular children referred to him were misdiagnosed.[65] He wrote that it was 'necessary to correlate the history of the case and the clinical findings with a tuberculin test, a sedimentation time and an X-ray'. The TOs in the Dublin area rarely used tuberculin tests, according to Collis. This was due to 'lack of proper paediatric training of students in our medical schools'. More positively, a state-funded initiative in 1945, in the form of the Dublin Corporation Primary Tuberculosis Clinic, provided a locus of best practice with respect to childhood tuberculosis. This was the 'first attempt by any local authority in these islands to set up a medical centre for the special study and control of primary tuberculosis in children', according to Mairead Dunlevy, the medical officer in charge of the clinic.[66] In Great Britain, the need for engagement by the public health service with childhood tuberculosis was disputed by the British Paediatric Association, which was in favour of such engagement, and the Tuberculosis Association, which was against it. The latter association stated that childhood tuberculosis was 'not of great importance' to public health and urged paediatricians to 'preserve a sense of proportion'.[67] This tussle might also be read in terms of paediatricians asserting the need for separate treatment of children and, hence, the need for their specialism to develop along separate lines to adult medicine.

MAPPING TUBERCULOSIS IN IRISH CHILDREN

While tuberculin was useful for diagnosis of tuberculosis in individual children, the publication of studies with respect to the tuberculin status of Irish children living in various environments provided epidemiological maps of the changing patterns of childhood tuberculosis between 1930 and 1950. In 1934, Price reported on the results of tuberculin testing of 500 children attending Dublin hospitals.[68] This survey demonstrated the low rate of tuberculin positivity among these children compared with children in Lund, Sweden and Helsinki, Finland. In 1933, Price tuberculin tested fifty healthy girls and five boys, in the 14 to 18 age category, attending Coláiste Móibhí, Dublin, a preparatory school for trainee teachers, where she was the medical officer. The big surprise with the overall results of the survey was the low rate of positivity among the adolescents, indicating they had not been previously exposed to tuberculosis and, therefore, had no immunity.[69] This study was important in that it disproved the belief among the medical profession that healthy young Irish adults had all been exposed to tuberculosis. Price later extended this work over an eleven-year period, publishing results in 1939 and 1945.[70] The pattern of low positivity was borne out in later, more extensive tuberculin studies, with lower rates in rural than urban areas. In 1938, the

Irish Paediatric Association, at Price's instigation, undertook a tuberculin survey among sick children attending hospitals in Dublin. This survey of more than 1,000 children demonstrated that many cases of tuberculosis would have been misdiagnosed in the absence of a tuberculin test.[71] In 1945, Patricia Alston, an assistant physician at St Ultan's who worked alongside Price, carried out a study of various forms of diagnostic tuberculin skin tests in Artane Industrial School, Dublin. This study, which attested to the value of Dublin Moro, identified five hitherto undiagnosed cases of tuberculosis among the boys incarcerated in the school.[72] In 1946, T.M. Kavanagh of the Children's Hospital, Temple Street, Dublin reported on the tuberculin testing of children attending the medical outpatients. Of 1,330 children tested, 371 reacted positively to tuberculin, providing further proof of the low rates of immunity against tuberculosis among Irish children.

Patrick Fitzpatrick, Deputy CMOH in Cork city, showed how tuberculin testing could be used to trace children who had been exposed to tuberculosis. When an 8-year-old school child presented with tuberculosis, it was decided to examine the thirty-eight children in the class. All tested positive with tuberculin and Fitzpatrick theorized that this was because of contact with the infected child. It was 'more than probable' that many schools had latent cases of re-infection tuberculosis. He suggested that an attempt should be made to find and segregate these cases as the danger from them was apparent.[73] From 1944 to 1946, the Anti-Tuberculosis section of the Irish Red Cross carried out a survey of children and young adults attending primary schools, industrial schools and orphanages in Cork city and suburbs.[74] A much higher incidence of tubercular infection was found among girls than boys. This extensive study of more than 7,300 children found that two-thirds of the cohort reacted positively to tuberculin. According to Fitzpatrick, this deviation from the lower rates reported elsewhere in Ireland represented 'widespread uncontrolled dissemination of infection'.[75] Fitzpatrick used the data produced by this study to call for a 'systematic search' for cases, showing how epidemiology could feed back into individual diagnosis as well as feeding forward into producing a map of tuberculosis exposure. In Great Britain, the skin test was assuming greater importance in the search for tubercular children, with Wilfrid Gaisford, physician to the Warwickshire County Hospitals, asserting in 1946 that it was the 'only sure diagnostic test'.[76] However, the Chief TO of London City Council, Frederick Heaf, noted that paediatricians were inclined to think treatment was necessary in all children with a positive skin test and an abnormal shadow in the lungs, while general practitioners were reluctant to send the child away unless there were definite symptoms.[77] In Price's view, every child was either infected or not. For her, a positive skin test indicated infection, which could then be evaluated in the light of radiological and clinical findings.[78]

At national level in Ireland, tuberculosis began to assume an importance it had not previously been accorded. According to Greta Jones, the treatment of tuberculosis left behind the 'despair and futility' which characterized it in the 1920s and 1930s and, in the mid-1940s, took on 'an iconic significance in the push for social reform'.[79] The increased mortality from tuberculosis in Ireland during the Second World War, the appointment of James Deeny as chief medical adviser, the White Paper on tuberculosis in 1946, the creation of a separate Department of Health in 1947, Ireland's first inter-party government in 1948, and the appointment of Noel Browne as Minister for Health, along with the lengthy drafting and implementation of the 1947 Health Act, which had its genesis in 1944, combined to push an agenda that included provision of additional hospital beds, and preventative and support measures to tackle tuberculosis. Browne appointed Price to chair the statutory Consultative Council on Tuberculosis, which had an advisory function with respect to national anti-tuberculosis policy. Relying on the evidence of epidemiological surveys, particularly those highlighting the tuberculin status of Irish children and rural adolescents, as well as international data, Price urged the establishment of a national BCG vaccination programme.[80] In 1949 she was appointed as the first chairperson of the newly established National BCG Committee. A paediatrician was now leading two major anti-tuberculosis initiatives in Ireland.

By the 1950s the overall death rate from tuberculosis in Ireland was significantly higher than in neighbouring countries, with 0.8 deaths per 1,000 population in Ireland compared to 0.48 in Northern Ireland, 0.36 in England and Wales and 0.34 in Scotland. By the end of the 1950s the Irish death rate from tuberculosis had fallen but it was still almost twice the rate in Great Britain, with 0.2 deaths per 1,000 population in Ireland in 1958, 0.11 in Northern Ireland, 0.10 in England and Wales and 0.13 in Scotland.[81] In 1952 Price collated the results of 10,000 tuberculin reactions carried out by the National BCG Committee. These included 'every age-group, from infancy to 50 years, and persons in every walk of life and all income groups'.[82] Less than 7 per cent of children up to the age of 4 years had a positive tuberculin reaction, demonstrating that they had not been exposed to tuberculosis and had no acquired immunity. Throughout the 1950s, tuberculin testing continued to be used as a warning mechanism, a sort of crude predictor of remaining infection in the community. Tuberculin testing of primary school children in Dublin in the 10 to 14-year-old age group, carried out in 1957, found the percentage of positive reactions was high. At 43 per cent it was similar to the 1947 figure and much higher than corresponding rates in Britain and Northern Ireland in the late 1950s. At the same time, clinically significant tuberculosis rates in Dublin, detected using mass radiography, were higher than corresponding rates in Northern Ireland, although Mairead Dunlevy concluded that the 'present picture of childhood tuberculosis' in Dublin was remarkably 'satisfactory'.[83] A later study found that almost one third of Dublin teenagers, tested at age 13 at the end of 1961, reacted positively to tuberculin, compared to less than 1 per cent in rural areas.[84] Tuberculin testing served to point out the continuing presence of *Mycobacterium tuberculosis* in the Irish capital.

CONCLUSIONS

Childhood tuberculosis and the difficulties in diagnosing this disease in children have received scant attention in the historiography of tuberculosis in twentieth-century Ireland. This chapter has demonstrated that the patchy engagement with one useful diagnostic test, the tuberculin test, by the Irish medical profession up until the late 1940s is deserving of further attention as it had serious implications for individual Irish children and for policy development with respect to tuberculosis. Caution among the Irish medical profession with respect to the test may have been due to reservations expressed in the British medical journals for the first four decades of the twentieth century. This chapter has shown that the tuberculin test was introduced to Ireland through a network of connections between Irish and continental – primarily Scandinavian – paediatricians, subverting the usual model whereby the Irish medical profession looked to Great Britain.

In both Great Britain and Ireland, the increased focus on childhood tuberculosis rendered paediatricians and their work visible and provided validity for the continuing development of paediatrics as a separate specialism. The paediatricians Robert Collis and Dorothy Price were active in highlighting the problem of childhood tuberculosis and in promoting the use of the tuberculin test, and were founding members of the Irish Paediatric Club. Price's chairmanship of the Consultative Council on Tuberculosis and the National BCG Committee ensured paediatrics and childhood tuberculosis were visible in Ireland at national level.

In addition to its role in the diagnosis of childhood tuberculosis, tuberculin testing was useful in mapping tuberculosis infection in Irish children in the middle third of the twentieth century when mortality and morbidity remained relatively high. Anne Hardy has posited that perceptions of tuberculosis changed in Great Britain following a series of epidemiological studies carried out between 1940 and 1970. This chapter has applied Hardy's thesis to childhood tuberculosis in Ireland and demonstrated that childhood tuberculosis was reconceptualized in Ireland in a similar manner, with epidemiological studies of patterns of tuberculosis infection in Irish children commencing in the 1930s. The belief held by the medical profession that all Irish children had been exposed to tuberculosis – usually due to the ingestion of infected milk or by respiratory inspiration of the tubercle bacillus – by the time they reached adolescence was shown to be untrue. A proportion of

Irish children, particularly those who were raised in rural areas, remained tuberculin negative into their late teens. This meant that they had not been exposed to tuberculosis and remained susceptible to infection, providing the rationale for a national preventive vaccination strategy. However, the contribution of various iatrogenic interventions, such as vaccination, to the fall in tuberculosis mortality and morbidity has been vigorously debated.

Its contribution to the decline in tuberculosis notwithstanding, the introduction of mass vaccination has caused the tuberculin test to lose its value with respect to population studies in Great Britain and Ireland. In the United States, where mass vaccination against tuberculosis was not instituted, the tuberculin test is still of use in epidemiological studies.[85] Tuberculin is still used in Ireland for individual diagnosis and for tracing contacts of actively infectious tubercular patients. The current national guidelines on the prevention and control of tuberculosis in Ireland state that there is no 'gold standard for determining whether a person is infected with *Mycobacterium tuberculosis*, but, in practice, the tuberculin skin test is the standard method used'.[86] Tuberculin testing may also be used to trace persons who have been in contact with tuberculosis in situations such as the outbreak in 2010 among children attending a school in Cork.[87]

8

Rickets and Irish Children: Dr Ella Webb and the Early Work of the Children's Sunshine Home, 1925–1946[1]

Laura Kelly

From the 1920s to the 1940s, rickets was publicized in the Irish press as being a serious health concern.[2] Although national figures for rickets in Ireland in the 1920s and 1930s do not exist, the incidence of rickets among children in Dublin in the year 1939–40, based on the records of the radiological departments of children's hospitals, was reported to be 10 per 1,000 and in 1941–2 the incidence had doubled to 23 per 1,000.[3] Professor W.E. Jessop, chairman of the Nutritional Council of the Irish Medical Association for the Irish National Nutrition Survey, undertook a study of the prevalence of rickets among Dublin children between 1942 and 1948.[4] During the spring months of these years, Jessop surveyed samples of child patients at three children's hospitals and one welfare centre. He reported that the incidence of rickets in Dublin was 173 per 1,000 children in 1943.[5] Wartime restrictions on imported wheat made it essential to increase the extraction rate of flour between September 1940 and February 1942, which had an adverse effect on calcium absorption and increased the incidence of rickets. Additionally, in this period, the importation of cod liver oil and other concentrated sources of Vitamin D had greatly fallen as a result of the war.[6] The incidences decreased to 96 per 1,000 in 1945, when the extraction rate of flour had been reduced to 85 per cent.[7]

This chapter will explore the early efforts of one institution – the Children's Sunshine Home in Stillorgan, Dublin – which was founded by Dr Ella Webb, an Irish doctor, in 1925 to manage the disease.[8] The chapter suggests that Webb's work may be situated as part of a scheme of philanthropic social work conducted by a network of Irish women doctors in Dublin that particularly focused on women and children.[9] As Jacinta Prunty has argued, charitable institutions in Dublin in the nineteenth and twentieth centuries 'played an important role in the alleviation of daily hardships' experienced by the dwellers of Dublin's slums, particularly when set against the backdrop of limited state provision.[10] The Children's Sunshine Home was distinctive in that, unlike many other charitable institutions from the period, it was founded on non-sectarian lines.[11] Despite the lack of proselytism, there is evidence to suggest that the home served the function of 'improving' the lower-class children of Dublin's slums and moulding them into efficient members of the nation.[12]

Rickets is a childhood disease caused by a lack of Vitamin D. Vitamin D is required by the body for the absorption of calcium and phosphorus, thus without Vitamin D the body cannot properly build bones. The disease was first described by Francis Glisson, a British physician, in the seventeenth century and became common in northern Europe and North America in the nineteenth and early twentieth centuries, in particular among the urban poor.[13] Industrial towns were breeding grounds for rickets, which became widely known as 'the English disease'.[14] The disease also had a seasonal pattern and cases were most numerous during the spring months.[15] In Ireland, the primary causes attributed to rickets were over-crowded, ill-ventilated homes and a lack of exercise and proper food. Dublin will be the focus of this chapter because it is both the area from which the patients of the Children's Sunshine Home came, and also where the condition appears to have been most prevalent. Children suffering from rickets developed soft and elastic bones and, if nothing was done, deformity soon followed.[16] In Dublin, many poor families within the inner city were housed in tenements that were essentially large, vacated Georgian houses that had been converted into accommodation for poorer families.[17] According to Prunty, 'condemnation of appalling sanitary conditions, overcrowding and excessive mortality was often accompanied by generalized references to the real or presumed immorality and ignorance festering therein'.[18] Furthermore, as Mary E. Daly has shown, social class was the most important determinant of children's health, with the child mortality rate for children aged between 1 and 5 of hawkers, labourers and porters being 12.7 per 1,000 in contrast to 0.9 per 1,000 of the professional classes.[19]

The diet of the poor in Dublin was also significantly deficient, with evidence suggesting that, 'at least until the 1950s, the diet and nutrition of the average poor or working-class family was substandard'.[20] Investigations into the diet of the poor in Dublin in the twentieth century revealed a heavy dependence on bread and tea and very limited consumption of meat and vegetables.[21] Evidently, poor diet and housing had a negative impact on the health of those living in the tenements. One Englishman visiting Dublin in 1917 commented that the poor of Dublin were often stunted in growth and appeared 'deformed and misshapen'.[22] One former inhabitant of an early twentieth-century Dublin tenement remarked that around Gardiner Street these characteristics were readily observable among the poor but were little understood at the time: 'Looking back on it now and seeing the children of today, they were so *undersized* and very thin. Their little legs were like matchsticks. And a lot of children in those days suffered rickets and were bow-legged. We thought they were born that way but they weren't, it was malnutrition, they hadn't the vitamins.'[23] Another man who grew up in Dublin's tenements, Patrick O'Leary, commented that 'a lot of their [the inhabitants of the tenements'] illnesses were born of the fact that they weren't properly nourished. Their diet was bread, margarine and tea.'[24] Such comments suggest that poor living conditions and diet were recognized as contributing to a variety of illnesses, one of which was rickets. Moreover, these observations signify the prominence of the issue of securing healthy childhood growth in the period. Childhood became reconceptualized and, as shown in the work of Édouard Séguin, a French physician and educationist, and Margaret MacMillan, a British educationist and socialist propagandist, the belief existed that 'working-class children could be rescued from deprived circumstances, made whole, well and strong, and educated to become agents of a new social future'.[25]

The health problems of children living in Dublin's tenements did not go unnoticed by the medical profession. In 1926 the eminent British orthopaedic surgeon Sir Robert Jones visited Dublin and gave addresses at several meetings relating to the problem of crippled children in Ireland. Jones estimated that there were approximately 12,000 to 14,000 crippled children in Ireland, the chief diseases causing crippling being tuberculosis and rickets. Jones also commented on the appalling conditions of the Dublin hospitals, stating that although the work done there was 'absolutely splendid, the conditions under which the surgeons in them worked were [sic] really almost pathetic'.[26] Similarly, Dr Dorothy Stopford Price, who is discussed in Anne Mac Lellan's chapter in this volume, wrote in 1958 that it was through Webb's work in the outpatients department of the Adelaide Hospital, and in St Ultan's Hospital, that Webb came to realize that there were few beds available for children under 5 years suffering from rickets.[27] Although children with rickets were also treated at Cappagh House, a convalescent home for children suffering from tuberculosis, rickets and malnutrition that was founded by the Sisters of Charity in 1921, and at the Cheeverstown Convalescent Home, founded in 1904, Webb argued that 'none of the existing institutions are available for cases of this kind', with the former 'always filled with convalescent operation cases from Temple Street Hospital' and the latter '[which] cannot deal with children unable to run about'. She and her committee believed that the Children's Sunshine Home would allow the provision of open-air and 'appropriate treatment' exclusively for children suffering from rickets.[28]

IRISH WOMEN DOCTORS, PHILANTHROPY AND CHILD HEALTH AND WELFARE

Ella Webb (née Ovenden) (1877–1946) was the daughter of the Very Reverend Charles T. Ovenden, rector of Enniskillen and later Dean of St Patrick's.[29] She undertook her secondary education at Queen's College, Harley Street, London and at Alexandra College before entering the Catholic University of Ireland and graduating with a BA degree in 1899. Following this, she undertook a medical degree, graduating as MB (Bachelor of Medicine), BCh (Bachelor of Surgery), BAO (Bachelor of Obstetrics) in 1904 and MD (Doctor of Medicine) in 1906.[30] She won an RUI (Royal University of Ireland) travelling scholarship to Vienna in 1905, which she embarked upon the following year.[31] She married George Webb, a fellow of Trinity College Dublin, in 1907.[32] Webb worked as a demonstrator of physiology to women medical students at Trinity College Dublin and also at the Catholic University Medical School before being elected to the visiting staff of the Adelaide Hospital in Dublin.[33] She established a dispensary for children there in 1918.[34] Her chief interest throughout her career was the provision of medical care and treatment to children.[35]

Writing in 1907 on the position and career prospects of women doctors in Ireland, Webb commented:

> These prospects are improving every year, as the woman doctor takes a more established place in the community, but her position will only be secure as she shows that she has taken up medicine, not as a fad, but as a serious scientific or philanthropic undertaking.[36]

This quote illustrates Webb's firm belief in the Irish woman doctor's role in the community and suggests that she believed that women doctors would only succeed if they showed themselves to be serious about the philanthropic and scientific aspects of their work. Like many middle-class Protestant women of her time, Webb was heavily involved in such work during her lifetime. Philanthropy allowed middle- and upper-class women to become aware of the problems facing the working classes.[37] Maria Luddy has shown how Irish middle-class women, motivated by Christian duty, were heavily involved in charitable work in the nineteenth and twentieth centuries.[38] Additionally, Oonagh Walsh's extensive study of Anglican women in early twentieth-century Dublin has highlighted the 'significant and often unexpected contributions' that women of the Church of Ireland have made to the modern Irish state through philanthropic activities.[39] For example, Margaret Ó hÓgartaigh's work on Dr Kathleen Lynn has highlighted the role of women doctors, including Webb, in St Ultan's Hospital, which was founded by Lynn and Madeline ffrench-Mullen in 1919 in response to social conditions among the poor in Dublin.[40]

Several early Irish women doctors, like Webb, involved themselves in philanthropic work that complemented their medical careers. Elizabeth Tennant, who graduated from the Royal College of Surgeons in Ireland in 1894, worked as a medical officer to St Catherine's School and Orphanage in Dublin while also running a busy general practice in the city. She became a member of staff at St Ultan's Hospital from its foundation in 1919. Tennant's obituary claims that her 'keenness and energy put her on a level with her male colleagues'.[41] Some Irish women doctors also played a role in suffrage organizations. While campaigning for female suffrage, Webb also promoted policies relating to child welfare. She spoke at a meeting of the Irish Women's Reform League in 1914, urging the government to provide increased maternity benefits, schools for mothers and baby clinics.[42] Similarly, Emily Winifred Dickson, an 1891 graduate of the Royal College of Surgeons in Ireland, also recognized the potential for women doctors to contribute to Irish society, particularly in relation to issues concerning women and children. At a meeting of the Irish Suffrage Association in Dublin she urged 'the necessity of well-to-do women taking an interest in questions which affected working women'. She was also involved in the National Society for the Prevention of Cruelty to Children and the Irish Association for the Prevention of Intemperance and campaigned for the need for women as Poor Law guardians in Ireland and for a reform of the Irish workhouse system.[43]

Webb, as well as Katharine Maguire (who graduated through the Royal College of Science in 1891), Lily Baker (a 1906 graduate of Trinity College Dublin) and Prudence Gaffikin (who trained at Queen's College Belfast but qualified with the conjoint Scottish diploma in 1900), was actively involved in the Women's National Health Association (WNHA). A later graduate, Mabel Crawford (née Dobbin, Trinity College Dublin, 1913), acted as secretary to the Dublin University Mission in addition to playing a leading role in 'Baby Week', an event organized by the WNHA, the aim of which was to reduce infant mortality rates in Ireland.[44] The WNHA had been established by Lady Aberdeen, the wife of the lord lieutenant John Hamilton-Gordon, as a voluntary and charitable organization with the aim of improving maternity and child welfare in addition to helping to combat tuberculosis, Ireland's most serious health problem in the early twentieth century.[45]

Fundamentally, the WNHA had one major aim: 'to reach the women of the country' and to educate them about questions of health and sanitary medicine.[46] This was in keeping with contemporary middle-class notions that the mother was responsible for the survival of infants and the health of children and that in order to provide healthy future citizens for the nation, mothers needed to improve by becoming educated.[47] As Ó hÓgartaigh has shown, the WNHA and the committee of St Ultan's co-operated in the training of health visitors and in the education of mothers in child healthcare.[48] One of the main ways the WNHA tried to educate mothers was through its travelling exhibition in 1907, in which Webb played an active role. The exhibition visited between eighty and ninety places in Ireland and attracted large crowds.[49] Webb, along with Lily Baker, another Irish doctor, was placed in charge of the 'domestic science' display of the exhibition, which illustrates the organization's belief that facts relating to public health could be 'driven home better still by individual speaking to individual, by woman speaking to woman, by mother speaking to mother'.[50] Mothers were also targeted by advertisements in Irish newspapers for food supplements to prevent rickets.

For example, an advertisement for Jessel's cod liver extract tablets carried the headline 'Mother! Rickets can be prevented.'[51] Another advertisement for Scott's emulsion included a testimony from a mother who had given the product to her baby and noticed an improvement in one month.[52] Such advertisements, in line with their American counterparts, worked on several premises: firstly, suggesting that the mother was responsible for the health of her child; secondly, that 'dire consequences would arise unless the mother provided the child with the advertised product'; and thirdly, that the mother who did not buy the advertised product would be punished with a sick child.[53]

Furthermore, a letter from Reverend R.M. Gwynn (1877–1962) (a professor and fellow at Trinity College Dublin and one of the founders of the Dublin University Social Service Society) published in the *Irish Times* in 1931 highlights the responsibility given to Irish mothers for the health of their children as well as the issues facing Webb:

> Dr Ella Webb, whose Sunshine Home at Stillorgan is the salvation of so many children attacked by rickets, says that she could fill it over and over again from the dispensary which she runs for the infants of the poor. To many she can only say, 'Keep your child lying in the open air'. But how can a mother do this, who has only a room up three flights of stairs, and a fractional share in a tiny yard, insanitary because one lavatory and tap has to serve the whole house containing at least seven families?[54]

It was through her role as a paediatrician at the Infant Clinic at St Ultan's Hospital, and at the Adelaide Hospital, that Webb treated many cases of rickets. Writing in 1935, she remarked:

> In the year 1923, I was so much struck with the futility of my own treatment of rickets in the outpatient department of the Adelaide Hospital that I determined something must be done

about it. I was fortunate enough to arouse the interest and enlist the sympathy of a friend who was willing to give some financial assistance to the extent of £250 a year until we got established.[55]

The patients' homes were usually the dark, overcrowded tenement slums of Dublin. The conditions of these tenements were such that rickets and tuberculosis were commonplace and many of the patients had little hope of recovery following admission to hospital. Through ignorance and poverty, many of the patients were unable to follow the recommended treatment of diet and aftercare. It was against this background, and the apparent lack of adequate treatment for rickets patients in Irish hospitals, that Webb explored the possibility of finding a home to treat at least some of her patients.[56]

THE FOUNDATION OF THE CHILDREN'S SUNSHINE HOME

In her role as a volunteer with the St John Ambulance, Webb knew Letitia Overend, the Chief Staff Officer of the Women's Section, who was eager to help with the project of building an institution to care for children with rickets. Overend's uncle made a generous donation of £5,000 in 1923 towards the fund. With the help of some eager friends, Webb set about finding suitable premises for the home. She, and the other women who later made up the committee of the Children's Sunshine Home, inspected 'practically every vacant house in County Dublin' but decided that it would make more financial sense to build their own premises.[57] It was proposed that the house would not only be a centre of treatment but would also allow for the study of rickets.[58] In 1924 the Board of the Convalescent Home on Leopardstown Road offered to lease a field for the building of the home, and a wooden bungalow-type house with open verandahs was planned.[59]

The Children's Sunshine Home opened on St Patrick's Day, 1925 with room for twenty patients, but with a view to expansion.[60] It was erected at a total cost of £2,348, with an additional sum of £500 spent on equipment. There was an endowment of £250 per annum, but the rest of the expenses were dependent on voluntary contributions.[61] At a talk given by the Committee of Management and the Matron, Webb explained to a large audience the objects used by the home for the special treatment of rickets in young children. One attendee at the talk commented that 'the little patients in airy attire, disporting themselves in their sunbath on the lawn in front of the house, formed a picture at once interesting and appealing: the enthusiasm of their enjoyment seemed to communicate itself to the guests who unanimously expressed their appreciation of the afternoon function'.[62] There were regular fundraising efforts, including fetes and dances and performances of plays and music at various locations in Dublin. The home relied on public generosity and did not receive funding from the Irish Hospitals' Sweepstakes. Appeals were also regularly made in the press for public support.

One article in the *Dublin Evening Mail* commented on the dangers of rickets, stating that 'next to tuberculosis, there is scarcely any infantile complaint more insidious in its effects and destructive in its results. City children in particular are peculiarly subject to the disease, aggravated as it is by both environment and lack of suitable nourishment. It is probably one of the largest ramifications of misery endangered by the city milk supply'.[63] This comment draws attention to the problems of the Dublin milk supply in the 1920s. In 1924, the Rockefeller Foundation highlighted the poor hygiene practices of Irish dairies and creameries.[64] Furthermore, in 1928 the Inter-Departmental Committee on Dublin's Milk Supply found that 2.66 per cent of random samples taken of the capital's milk contained the tuberculosis bacillus. Additionally, of cows slaughtered in the Dublin area in 1926, 24 per cent showed evidence of tuberculosis.[65] The situation remained unchanged for over a decade until research undertaken by Cecil Mushatt under the supervision of J.W. Bigger's Pathology Laboratory at Trinity College Dublin discovered that over the period 1928 to 1929, about one third of the cows slaughtered in Dublin were tuberculous.[66] Webb was actively involved in efforts to regulate the Dublin milk supply and in 1910 published a report with Lily Baker, another Irish female doctor, on the Dublin Pasteurised Milk Depot, which had been established by the Women's National Health Association in 1908

– following a donation from the New York businessman and philanthropist Nathan Straus – to help combat the problem of infected milk.[67]

In addition to her publications in medical journals and campaigning for improvements in child and maternity welfare, Webb published numerous requests in the Irish press for donations towards the Children's Sunshine Home. In August 1924 she wrote to the *Irish Times* stating that the building of the home was near completion and requested monetary donations, in addition to promises of articles of equipment such as children's cots, furniture for the matrons' and staff rooms, bedding, linen, kitchen utensils and cleaning requisites.[68] The subscription lists of the Children's Sunshine Home are testament to the huge public support it received.[69] The emotive issue of sick children may have been responsible for the generous support pledged to the home, and the appeals for financial support frequently played on this issue. For example, a 1927 appeal included a startling quote from the honorary consulting surgeon to the home:

> Sir William Wheeler, the Hon. Consulting Surgeon writes: 'Can you make room for a surgical case – a child of three years old, having a broken leg, which will not knit without sunshine? The alternative is amputation.'[70]

Similarly, an appeal leaflet from 1925 for funding for equipment for the home ended with the question 'Can YOU deny the Children this chance?'[71] Another Christmas appeal envelope from 1924 asked 'Will you help these Children?'[72] Such questions may have touched the public and helped the home to raise donations.

The Children's Sunshine Home set out a detailed scheme upon its foundation. It established a Committee of Management that would undertake the management and administration of the home and be responsible for its direction. The first of these committees was comprised of twelve philanthropic women.[73] It was agreed that the home was founded 'for the care and treatment of children suffering from weak or misshapen limbs, and from the ailment commonly known as Rickets, and other ailments of a similar character' and that the home would be open to both boys and girls under the age of 8. These children would be provided with medical and surgical treatment and, where necessary, with surgical appliances. It was also decided that the home would be open to 'all suffering children, irrespective of the religious faith to which they belong' and that all patients, officials, nurses and servants connected with the home would be afforded every facility to practise their religion without any interference.[74] Similarly, in its May 1925 appeal it was stated that the home was run 'on absolutely non-sectarian lines'.[75] This suggests that the home was aware of the public's fears of proselytism. Lindsey Earner-Byrne has highlighted the fear of proselytism in twentieth-century Ireland, which meant that Protestant or non-sectarian charities were suspected of being 'only interested in helping Catholics in order to convert them'.[76] Related to this, Ó hÓgartaigh's research has shown how Dr Kathleen Lynn's work 'brought her into conflict with the Catholic Church, which closely monitored the activities of philanthropic organizations'.[77] Moreover, St Ultan's Hospital faced particular difficulties with regard to the question of its Protestant management, which arose during negotiations for the amalgamation of St Ultan's with the National Children's Hospital at Harcourt Street.[78] I have not found evidence that the Children's Sunshine Home experienced similar problems, despite the fact that its committee was also largely comprised of Protestant women. Revealingly, in 1942 permission was granted to the Nursery Rescue Society and the Catholic Protection Society (a society that particularly targeted families and children threatened by proselytism),[79] which were both experiencing financial difficulties, to send children to the home free of charge.[80] This suggests that the home was not seen as an agent of proselytism.

'A CHANCE TO BECOME A HEALTHY AND USEFUL CITIZEN': THE WORK OF THE CHILDREN'S SUNSHINE HOME

The Children's Sunshine Home was a philanthropic organisation that facilitated the treatment of a disease which, at the time of the home's foundation, was not, in Webb's eyes, being adequately treated by Irish hospitals. The following table indicates the numbers of patients admitted in the period, which fluctuated over time. In 1928 forty-six patients were admitted, with thirty-one discharged cured and three discharged improved. In 1935 the home admitted ninety-seven children during the year; fifty-nine were discharged cured and eight improved. The average length of residence in this year was ninety-six days. The increase in the number of patients admitted is likely to have been as a result of the extensions made to the institution in the 1930s, when a new ward was added. Furthermore, writing in 1935, Webb also pointed out that there had been great improvements in child welfare administration in the city and that there had been a gradual awakening of the public to the possibility of a cure, which demonstrated a shift from earlier beliefs articulated by parents to Webb that 'God made the child's legs that way and it was not for me to interfere'.[81] This may also partly account for the high number of patients admitted during the 1930s. Webb additionally acknowledged that there had been improvements in the supply of fresh, clean milk to the poor and in housing conditions.[82]

The numbers of patients discharged cured remained consistently high throughout the period. After 1944, the number of patients admitted began to decrease again. This may have been partly as a result of the reduction of the extraction rate of flour, which was reduced from wartime levels of 100 down to 85 per cent, resulting in a decrease in incidence of rickets in children. Following the fortification of bakers' flour with acid calcium-phosphate, the incidence of rickets fell even further.[83]

The work of the Sunshine Home received positive recognition from patients' parents following their discharge. For example, in 1927 Mrs D., the mother of a child, Kathleen, who had been a patient in the home, wrote to Letitia Overend on the committee of the Children's Sunshine Home to say:

> Dear Madam, I beg to inform you that I have my daughter Kathleen home again. She is in splendid health and we are very pleased with the result of the treatment she received and are sure it will be a lasting benefit to her. I thank you very much for

Table 6. Figures for Patients Admitted to the Children's Sunshine Home, 1928-46*

Year	Number of patients admitted	Number of patients discharged cured	Number of cases discharged improved	Number of cases discharged no improvement	Number of cases transferred to hospital	Number of cases removed for various causes+
1928-29	46	31	3	0	2	4
1929-30	36	25	5	0	4	3
1930-31	45	32	4	1	3	4
1931-32	73	37	2	3	10	9
1934-35	67	17	6	3	16	8
1935-36	97	59	8	0	20	4
1936-37	75	46	8	2	16	5
1937-38	90	64	5	1	8	10
1940-41	65	38	9	1	17	1
1941-42	62	39	7	1	21	3
1942-43	78	47	10	0	11	0
1943-44	72	61	3	2	6	1
1944-45	58	34	3	0	20	1
1945-46	51	35	2	0	12	2

Source: Annual Reports of the Children's Sunshine Home (Overend Archive, Airfield Trust, Dublin).
* The figures for 1932-33, 1933-34 and 1938-39 and 1939-40 were not printed in the annual reports.
+ In the 1928-29 Annual Report for the Children's Sunshine Home, it is stated that such removals are 'sometimes due to parents leaving Dublin'.

your great kindness and for the interest you have taken in her, and to inform you that as soon as I am alright myself, I won't forget the Sunshine Home.[84]

Similarly, a letter was published in the 1937 annual report from J. and K.B. addressed to the secretary of the Children's Sunshine Home, Miss Moore, which thanked her for the help she 'rendered in getting Betty into the Sunshine Home' and remarked that the parents had 'not had the slightest trouble with her' since she returned home and that she had been 'wonderfully treated' at the institution.[85]

Webb's connection with the home also enabled her to undertake scientific research, for example on calcium metabolism in relation to disease.[86] Similarly, she participated in meetings at the Royal Academy of Medicine in Ireland. At one meeting of the section of State Medicine in 1935 on the topic of 'Some problems of public health', she commented on 'the delay on the part of mothers in seeking skilled aid for their ailing children'.[87] During the Second World War she created a formula and wrote a paper on the preparation of hips. According to her colleague Price, 'this was responsible for a campaign against scurvy and for the provision of free Vitamin C tablets by the Health Authority in Dublin'.[88] Similarly, the Committee of the Children's Sunshine Home played an active role in petitioning the government to ensure the regulation of the Dublin milk supply. In 1930 the Committee of Management of the Children's Sunshine Home passed a resolution stating that they would 'press earnestly upon the Government that immediate legislation was necessary to ensure that no contaminated milk should be sold in the Saorstát'. The committee believed that the 'present uncontrolled supply endangers the health of the children and is responsible for the widespread incidence of osseous tuberculosis'.[89] By this stage, in the 1930s, some of Dublin's milk was still found to contain unacceptable levels of bacteria.[90] However, research conducted by Joseph Bigger found that while only 2 per cent of Dublin milk was of certified standard in 1919/20, this had risen to 31 per cent in 1926/7 and to 62 per cent in 1932/3. Moreover, the number of tuberculin-tested herds around Dublin had risen from one to sixteen.[91]

The treatments conducted in the Children's Sunshine Home reflect contemporary understandings of rickets. Medical practitioners and researchers in the period were debating the relative importance of sunlight and vitamins in the treatment of the disease.[92] Fresh air and sunshine were an integral part of the treatment at the home, complemented by a diet rich in Vitamin D. Moreover, the location of the home, 'outside the smoke area, where the maximum of light and mountain air can be obtained', reflects contemporary emphasis on escape from the urban environment for the promotion of health, which can be traced back to the nineteenth century.[93] For rickets in the acute stage, the patient was kept entirely in bed and put on a full diet rich in Vitamin D, and given as much fresh air and sunshine as possible, the latter being supplemented in winter by the sunshine lamp. Cases of this kind generally lost all signs and symptoms of rickets in about four months, and if X-rayed in about six months showed definite signs of bony repair. Once bony repair was established, children were allowed to get up and play outside for a short time each day. For cases where bone deformities had already developed, the child was kept in bed without sunshine on a comparatively vitamin-poor diet for a short time while manipulation and splinting were proceeded with as briskly as possible. Once the bones had hardened, the child was put on the ordinary regimen. For the most severe cases, where deformities existed in apparently hard bones, the children were sent for surgical treatment in Mercer's Hospital and returned to the home when they were in plaster. Unless the weather was very wet and cold, or a child had some respiratory inflammation, patients remained out of doors on the verandah most of the day and all day and night in summer. They had two warm blankets each, a hot bottle and a warm jersey suit in winter, and according to Webb did 'not seem to feel cold'. The children were given a calcium-rich diet and regularly given cod liver oil with a high Vitamin D content.[94] The home was not without difficulties. Webb wrote that an outbreak of measles in 1933 meant that it had to close for two months. Similarly, in January 1934 the home closed for a few weeks due to an outbreak of diphtheria.[95]

Attendees at the annual meetings of the home often remarked positively on the good work that was being done there, and the reports on attendees highlight the link between the home and the Anglo-Irish gentry. For example, at the 1928 annual meeting the Earl of Wicklow commented that the institution was progressing favourably and that its finances were satisfactory. He commented that 'there was room in their country for more of that kind of work. They were trying to do something, but not in such a large way' for the treatment of children with rickets.[96] Another attendee, Her Excellency Mrs MacNeill, drew attention to the continued 'evil conditions' of cities like

Dublin, which 'often keep children, fresh air, and sunlight too far apart' and which she felt would take 'time and hard work to remove'.[97]

Within the annual reports and appeals of the Children's Sunshine Home, there is a sense that the committee believed that the home had important economic consequences and that there was an element of 'improving' the patients coming from the Dublin slums. In their 1925 letter of appeal, the committee stated: 'Sunshine and air are free to all, and it is sound national economy to prevent these children from filling up valuable space in hospitals and becoming burdens on the State.'[98] At the annual meeting in 1931, Dr Angela Russell commented that 'every child in the home had a chance to become a healthy and useful citizen', additionally remarking that 'the Sunshine Home helped to undo the harm which the slums had done'.[99] In their annual report in 1940, the board of the Children's Sunshine Home stated that 'the maintenance of an institution for the prevention and cure of ill health is one of the primary claims upon the liberality of thinking people'. Moreover, the report suggested that early attention to the health of children was an 'indispensable factor in the building up of the nation's life'.[100] The *Irish Press* reported: 'were it not for the Sunshine Home, many of the children, after being in hospital, would have had to go to their own homes, the condition of which often made recovery difficult. Children in the Sunshine Home got the best treatment and could be made efficient units of the population.'[101] Similarly, writing in 1953 about her twenty-eight years' association with the home, Price commented that 'many cases of Rickets have been cured completely, and many more have been so greatly improved that, with deformities corrected, they have grown into healthy useful citizens with a minimum stunting of growth'. Therefore, although the Sunshine Home did not proselytise, there is a sense that the committee and staff felt that the home had important economic consequences for the nation.

CONCLUSIONS

This chapter has outlined the work conducted by Dr Ella Webb in the early years of the Children's Sunshine Home. Although Webb herself died in 1946, the home continued to operate, and from the 1950s, with the decline in cases of rickets, it began to admit children suffering from diseases such as primary tuberculosis, coeliac disease and pre- and post-operative congenital heart disease, in addition to children in a debilitated state who required convalescence.[102] Webb's work in connection with the home is indicative of the emerging role of Irish women doctors in child welfare and philanthropy, while the case of rickets highlights how Irish mothers were deemed responsible for the health of their children. The home, unlike many other charitable institutions in the period, did not proselytize, yet there is a strong sense that it functioned, like many other charities involved in providing aid to inhabitants of Dublin's slums, in a period when state provision was limited.[103] Furthermore, despite not actively engaging in proselytism, it is evident that the staff of the home presented their work as providing an important economic function in turning child patients from the slums into 'useful citizens' and 'efficient units of the population'.[104]

9

THROUGH THE EYES OF A CHILD: 'SPANISH' INFLUENZA REMEMBERED BY SURVIVORS

Ida Milne

*I*n Ireland, the 1918–19 influenza pandemic is officially accredited with killing 20,057 people, and probably made more than 800,000 people ill.[1] The various estimates of global death from the disease suggest that it killed between 40 million and 100 million people, and infected between one fifth and half of the world's population, as it swept around the world in three or four waves over the two-year period, making it the largest of all known influenza pandemics.

This chapter draws on a collection of interviews with Irish child survivors of the pandemic. These interviews show that the epidemic made a lasting impact on the memories of children, despite the fact that they were not fully able to understand what was happening at the time. Some became curious listeners, trying to glean scraps of information about it from newspapers and from hushed adult conversations. For those who actually suffered from the disease, the event was frequently recalled as snapshots or scenes between the initial illness and the recovery as they drifted in and out of consciousness, in a febrile state. Most recovered, but for some, life or their health changed.

In Ireland this strain of influenza particularly affected two different age groups, the very young and young adults, the latter a group not normally badly affected by seasonal influenza.[2] Adults aged 25 to 35 accounted for 4,205 or 21 per cent of the Irish deaths certified to influenza from 1918 to 1919. Children under the age of 5 seemed to be particularly vulnerable to the disease, being far more likely to die from it than older children. Children aged 5 to 14 suffered the lowest death rate of any age group in comparison to the numbers living in their age sector. Of the 4,194 deaths of children under 15 certified to influenza in 1918 and 1919, 2,523 were younger than 5, or 12.5 per cent of the total certified influenza deaths.[3] In the 5 to 9 age group 905 children died, and in the 10 to 14 years age group 766 were certified as dying from influenza. These numbers ought to be viewed as conservative estimates of those who died from the disease for a variety of reasons. Some deaths were attributed to other causes, particularly in the early period of the epidemic, and there are reasonable grounds to suggest that many deaths were not recorded at all.[4]

What these statistics serve to illustrate is that this strain of influenza, by apparently singling out young adults and infants as its targets, affected young families. The statistics collected by the Irish registrar general do not permit an extrapolation of the numbers of children orphaned nor of the numbers of families that suffered multiple deaths. To acquire some concept of the enormous distress the disease caused those worst affected, we have to resort to checking through newspapers and to searching for personal accounts of families where the disease caused more than one death or where the death of one or both parents caused emotional trauma, severe economic hardship and even the dissolution of the family unit.

There appears to be a consensus among historians of the pandemic in other regions who have used oral testimony or memoir as a source that this type of evidence enables insights into the effects of the disease that cannot be acquired from other sources. These sources permit historians to acquire evidence about the social impact of the disease, how it affected individuals, families and communities in the short and long term, and how it was perceived or construed by ordinary people rather than how it was articulated in newspapers, official documents and institutional records. Apart from enabling an understanding of the direct impact on families, using oral history to study how a society responded, or was perceived to have responded, to major epidemics of disease can suggest interesting lines of inquiry. Robert A. Aronowitz has argued that the study of the effects of a disease on society is a useful exercise for the historian as disease can often evoke and reflect collective responses. Studying disease can provide an understanding of the values and attitudes of the society in which it occurs.[5] The Spanish influenza pandemic is a disease replete with social meaning. In an international context, that social meaning is loaded by its association with the First World War, while in an Irish context it is further complicated by association with key incidents in the revolutionary period, and with political tensions over governance and public attitude towards the key organs of state, in particular the Local Government Board (LGB), which bore responsibility for public health and sanitation.[6] The flu was, at once, one more trauma inflicted on society by the World War, and an aggravating factor that cast a magnifying glass over the British government's arguably key interaction with the Irish population – the provision of healthcare and welfare by the Local Government Board. Interviewing people about the impact of the pandemic on individuals and small groups facilitates an exploration of attitudes towards elements of the LGB's work – in particular the operation of the Poor Law medical system – as well as permitting an exploration of personal attitudes to, and conceptualizations of, Spanish influenza.

THE SAMPLE AND METHODS

When the idea of collecting interviews was first mooted as part of this author's doctoral research on the social history of the 1918–19 influenza pandemic in Leinster in autumn 2006, the epidemic was at a remove of eighty-eight years. While a scientific sampling did not seem possible, there were still many people alive who had lived through that time as children. The difficulty was to find them and, having found people who were willing to be interviewed, to find reliable witnesses. The first interviewees were acquired through personal contacts; others were contacted by telephoning nursing homes, through interviews on regional and national radio and articles in regional and national newspapers and in publications aimed specifically at the elderly. Eventually, as the project became better known and as news stories about the threats posed by avian and the 2009 H1N1 Influenza A or 'Mexican' flu stimulated interest in, and memory of, this last great influenza pandemic, people volunteered to participate. Some participated in formal, digitally recorded interviews; others, sometimes because of reticence, distance, or because they had not much to impart, were interviewed by telephone or through written communication. Over fifty influenza interviews were collected.[7]

The methods of oral historians are complex; one has to learn interviewing techniques, to read people, to listen with care and to interpret silences. Joanna Bornat has written of the need for the interviewer to understand the effect the interview has on the interviewee.[8] When interviewing about a traumatic episode such as Spanish influenza, the remembering can produce emotions that are difficult for both the interviewee and the interviewer to handle. Difficult, heavily considered passages of speech, long silences and outbursts of long-forgotten emotion are commonplace. Some of the interviews came to an abrupt end as the interviewees became overwhelmed by the emotion triggered by retrieving family or community tragedies from long-term memory. Some interviewees later suggested that the interviews were in some way cathartic, enabling them to make sense of an event which they had previously seen as an isolated episode of their childhood, allowing them to place it within the context of the pandemic and a wider catastrophe. Charles Rosenberg has argued that most people seek rational understanding of threatening epidemics to minimize their sense of vulnerability; some of these interviewees have lived another ninety years before being able to conceptualize their personal experience of Spanish flu in the wider framework of the disease.[9]

Everybody using oral history as a method faces a set of concerns peculiar to their own work as well as the issues common to all. In the case of oral histories of the Spanish flu, there are particular issues about age and memory. The subjects who had direct experience of the pandemic were born before 1918; the youngest was born in 1916, the oldest in 1903. Even without taking into account their current physiological condition or age-related brain degeneration, they were being asked to retrieve a memory that occurred ninety years before; a memory of something that happened when they were small children with underdeveloped language, deductive or analytical skills. Dealing with people in their 90s and 100s requires careful handling and some intuitive work. One may have to revert to the social mores of a different era to get the best out of them. They may need to be reassured that the interview is not a memory test, that they may not remember something like the 1918–19 influenza because it was outside their realm of experience; it might not have happened in their area, or might not have been spoken about in front of children.

THE INTERVIEWS

R.B. McDowell, former Junior Dean at Trinity College Dublin, came from a comfortably off Belfast family. He was 5 when he caught the flu in October 1918; the doctor was called and told his family that their little boy was unlikely to last the night. The doctor managed to get a private nurse to take care of the McDowell family, even though there was an extreme shortage of nurses because so many were serving at war. He survived, but could not recall what happened during the three weeks of his illness.[10] He was considered a delicate child for a long time after, which he described as having 'a mixed effect' on his character:

> It probably had the effect of weakening my resolution for hard work, you could always plead bad health. I was able up to the age of 12 or 14 to claim that I was an invalid, if school was too boring I could stay away. I think I expected a fair amount of indulgence, and could always get my own way, which inspires confidence … It certainly probably had at the back of my mind

that the army was out, because of bad health, and, should I go
to the bar, could I put up with the strain of being a barrister?

McDowell had heard that good nursing was the only real remedy, and offered
the opinion that as most middle-class households had a maid, and would
have had easy access to doctors and possibly been able to acquire a private
nurse, home nursing was possible and access to hospital was not a priority. He
pointed out that even for those in less fortunate circumstances hospitals did
not have the same priority as they would now, and that anyhow working-class
families might have considered going to the workhouse hospital 'as the end,
as a risk'.[11] The pandemic completely overburdened the Poor Law dispensary
system, which provided medical care for an estimated 70 per cent of the
population. The system was already experiencing staff shortages because
of an embargo on appointing doctors of an age to serve in the war. During
the pandemic, boards of guardians were constantly reporting difficulties in
appointing locum tenens to replace doctors who succumbed to the influenza;
many doctors worked around the clock to cope with the vast numbers of ill
seeking treatment, and some paid for their diligence with their lives.[12]

The view that flu sufferers in Belfast might regard entering the workhouse
hospital as risky was echoed in another interview, with veteran Belfast
journalist James Kelly, born in 1911, who said that people he knew who
were suffering from the flu were extremely reluctant to go to the workhouse
infirmary [now Belfast City Hospital] for treatment. 'Poor people did not
want it to be noted that they died in the Union.' He had heard that all the
hospitals in Belfast were packed out. His family lived on the Falls Road, which
was on the route to two cemeteries, and he spoke of 'black Belgian horses
pulling hearses for days going to the hospitals with more cabs following them'.
Kelly's grandmother and aunt died from the disease. Although admired by
his colleagues for his skills as a raconteur, the influenza epidemic had not
evolved into one of his renowned anecdotes. He was clearly distressed that
he could retrieve little else from this childhood memory other than that the
schools were closed.

Some child witnesses had exceptionally clear memories of the epidemic. Elizabeth Molloy was 97 when interviewed in February 2007, and had lived in the Dublin satellite town of Lucan all her life. She remembered feeling scared and isolated when all her five siblings and parents fell ill with the flu; the house was cold, there was no food; she heard 'the ching of spurs coming to the door', and knew that help was at hand. It was her uncle – she called him a 'horse soldier' – returning from the war. He put her to bed on the settle, and when she woke he had lit the fire, made a stew, and was busy doling out quinine and whiskey to her sick family. They all recovered. Most of them lived into their 90s, so flu clearly had no effect on their life expectancy. Soon afterwards, a neighbour's 12-year-old daughter died, a young girl who had been a ministering angel to Elizabeth's family and other neighbours bringing them food and supplies, until she too became ill. Elizabeth's words painted a vivid picture of the girl's distraught mother carrying the girl's body along the banks of the Grand Canal beseeching God to give her back.[13]

Mrs Molloy's story was clearly very well polished. She had been a shopkeeper for many years, and several people acquainted with her told me I should interview her, as they had heard her story. R.B. McDowell too has given an almost identical account to others, and even written it in his own memoirs; he was interviewed for a television documentary on personal experience of Spanish influenza and the material he used there was again almost identical to the interviews he gave to me.[14] Other interviewees spoke hesitatingly, reflecting in silences, as though it were the first time they had unearthed these memories of Spanish influenza since they had stored them in their long-term memory.

Catherine Doyle, 104 when interviewed, was clearly distressed by the memory of the flu, although she insisted that it had not been so bad in St Mullins, the County Carlow area where she lived at the time.[15] Born in 1903, she was 15 when the flu came. 'Oh, that black flu, that was a terrible thing, you'd never forget that,' she repeated several times. 'You'll have no trouble finding people to talk to you about that black flu.' It had made such an impression on her, when she heard there was at the time no Irish written history of the epidemic, she said: 'I am speechless.' She recalled her older brother Paddy getting it, and his 'lovely head of curls left on the pillow'. Hair loss was such a common feature of this influenza that newspaper advertisements offered products to remedy baldness caused by it. Paddy remained sickly for a long time afterwards. He was fed whatever he was able to take, usually gruel. She professed to being fascinated with Spanish flu because of her brother's experience with it.

> Oh, the people went black. I didn't see any of them but some of them did. Oh, but it was a desperate flu ... the poor curate, he was found at some crossroad one night, he had gone out, he was delirious. He got it and went out. You see, it was never too bad outside Dublin, Dublin was bad, the towns were bad but the country was fairly good. Two died from it in the parish. Just two. One was a train driver ... he went to fight it on his feet. There was no such thing as fighting that flu on your feet.[16]

Katie McMenamin caught the flu as a 14 year old, living in Rathmullan in County Donegal. She was 106 when contacted for this interview. She, her mother and three brothers and two sisters all caught it, but her father did not. Her mother brought it into their house, having gone to help nurse a neighbouring family who were all ill.

> My mother cared for us all while we were ill. I can remember that everyone with it complained of a terrible thirst and drank from jugs full of water. My youngest brother slept continuously for two full days without waking. Anyone prone to bronchitis or with a weak chest was likely to develop pneumonia from it and that usually proved fatal. My mother treated another of my brothers who had a weak chest by wrapping hot towels around his chest.[17]

She thought that Rathmullan's use as a naval base during the war might have been a factor in County Donegal having had an unusually high incidence of influenza in both 1918 and 1919. Many people in the village caught it and she was aware of several deaths, including four in one family. Like several other interviewees, she suggested that people did not talk about it afterwards because they dreaded the thought that it might come back again.

Olive Vaughan, née Burgess, was born in 1910 and lived in the south Dublin suburb of Donnybrook as a child. She was 8 at the time of the flu and was one of a family of eight children. She had overheard adults talking about people they knew having the flu, and hoping that they would be all right, and the next thing was that person would be dead.

> It seemed to sweep through the world, really. Everyone was frightened of it. It happened after the war. It was not forgotten in those days, I remember the horror.

Like R.B. McDowell, Mrs Vaughan said the emphasis of healthcare in those days was doctor-based. If people got sick, they called or visited a doctor rather than going to a hospital or a clinic. She could not recall her school being closed because of the epidemic. She expressed some surprise at not knowing more details about the flu, and considered that it might be because the adults in her family network used a type of code when they wanted to discuss things that were not considered appropriate for children to hear. This seems plausible as she could remember other contemporaneous events in detail.[18]

Enid [she asked to be referred to only by her first name] spoke of observing, as a 7 year old living in south Dublin, adults gathering in huddles to discuss this terrible illness that was going to kill more than were killed in the First World War. But when it did come, it did not affect her or anybody she knew. Like Mrs Vaughan, she suspected the reason she knew so little about the flu, despite having clear memories of other events at the time, was because her parents tried to prevent her hearing the more tragic stories. 'If there was tragedy the child might have been told to see if the kettle was boiling or something.'[19]

Some interviewees thought that either their access or lack of access to good-quality food had a bearing on the extent to which their family or community suffered from the flu. Tommy Christian considered good food to be a factor in his family's recuperation. 'We had our own vegetables and grand spring water; that was in our favour.' Tommy was born in 1913, and has lived all his life on the Boston Road in Ardclough, a rural community in north Kildare. As he spoke, he would leave long pauses, as he searched silently through the filing system of his memory. His mother, father, and he and his sister all got the flu.

> I was 5 years of age. We all got it, all the households, there was no one moving, even the doctor who was attending us got it. He was in Kill dispensary. The doctor had an old jalopy. He worked 24 hours round the clock on his own; he could come at three o'clock in the morning. Then he got it himself, and we were plastered altogether. We were stricken down for three weeks maybe, and recovering afterwards was the most trying time of it. [A long pause.] The health services weren't too good at the time. It was a terrible disaster.[20]

Tommy mentioned that there was a district nurse, but she was very old and only had a bicycle to travel on from Celbridge, four miles away. He said that all the businesses and shops in his area were closed, Masses suspended for a fortnight, and the landed estates were forced to hire women from the towns to do farm work.[21] Lyons Estate, seat of Lord Cloncurry, was across the road from Tommy's home; Lord Cloncurry's diary confirms that women from Celbridge were brought in to help with the farm work, because the flu had made the farm labourers ill. The Poor Law relieving officer, Mrs Byrne, came from Celbridge and gave them 'a few bob – about five shillings' to help them out, as his father, a self-employed cobbler, could not work during the flu. They sent word to her of their predicament and she came out to inspect them, and they got the money every week until his father was able to work again.[22]

> The descendants of those people living now, they don't know how lucky they are that their parents weren't swept away with it … [When asked about treatments for the flu he said] We were to make punch. We were to make sure that whatever you drank it was hot, the steam would help you, sure we could not swallow anything, our throats were so sore. And gruel, did you ever hear of gruel, it had an awful lot of responsibilities, this gruel. The O'Connors [a neighbouring farming family] brought us soup and stew, when they got back on their feet themselves … There wasn't a terrible lot of talk about it afterwards. They were afraid to talk about it in case they could get it again. But a terrible lot of bad chests resulted from it. I don't think we were the same again for a long time … it is a thing that will live with you for ever, that flu … Any survivors that got it would ever remember it. It was savage.[23]

Tommy Christian's mother died within a year of the epidemic. His father remarried, and moved to another house in the locality. Tommy and his sister were not part of the new household, remaining in their original home where an aunt cared for them. It was not until a subsequent interview that Tommy associated his mother's death as being caused by a *sequela* of influenza; she had never fully recovered her health after contracting the disease. This revelation was a surprise to the next generation of his family. Tommy's memory about other details relating to influenza in his locality has proven to have remarkable accuracy when cross-checked, so there seems little reason to doubt this association. There is no death certificate for Mrs Christian to confirm her cause of death. The absence of death certification has proven to be a common research finding in this study.

As this flu targeted young adults, Tommy's story of losing a parent and having family circumstances drastically changed by the flu is a common one. Nellie Tubridy, née Marrinan, was born prematurely in the spring of 1919 when her mother caught and died from influenza in Sligo, where her father was stationed with the Royal Irish Constabulary. Nellie weighed just over two pounds at birth and was given little chance of survival. She was assigned to the care of her father's sister, Ellen Corry, who lived with her husband and family at Churchtown, near Cooraclare in County Clare. The tiny infant was brought by train to Ennis, in a shoe box lined with cotton wool; from there, Ellen's husband John brought her to her new home by cart, resting at strategic intervals along the way in houses where he had arranged for fires to be lit, evidently aware that premature underweight babies face a particular risk of body heat loss. Ellen and John took it in turns to sleep on a settle by the fire with the baby until she was well enough to sleep alone. Nellie lived into her 80s, a bright and engaging woman who often told the story of her survival against the odds.[24]

Sometimes unearthing these memories from ninety years ago proved traumatic and almost as raw as if they had happened recently. Lena Higgins, born in Sallins, County Kildare in 1916, had been telling me of the trauma caused by the deaths of her father's two brothers who worked in shops in Arklow, when I mentioned the deaths of three children whose family owned a shop on Gorey's main street. These children turned out to be Lena's cousins, her father's two nephews and a niece. It is unclear whether she had associated their deaths with the flu before this interview, but the memory was too distressing to explore any further with her.[25]

Perhaps surprisingly, only one of the people interviewed for this research held the view that the disease was linked to perceptions of privations suffered by the Irish population as a result of oppression by the British imperialist system. Sister Theresa Connaghton, a Dominican nun, was born in 1912 on an island in Lough Reagh near Lanesboro, the eighth of ten children. She did not recall the flu happening at the time but was told about it later.[26]

My godmother, a neighbour, a young girl of 18, she died from the flu, I don't remember it. On the island, Inchéanaí, during the troubles, an old house was used as a hospital. I had a first cousin, they lived in County Roscommon, she died of the flu, 18 years of age. The country was very poor at that time, England had crushed them so much. The people were very poor and undernourished. It was no wonder that they all died.

Sister Wilfrid Callanan, born in 1916, believed this flu affected poor people worse than the better off. She lived in Patrickswell, County Limerick, with her family in a small house.

We were just after the big war, and there must have been an awful lot of shortages. Families were large. Six would be a small family. My mother spoke about the flu. I was only 2 years old in 1918 when the flu was raging. It took my uncle Paddy, my father's brother, and many others too. I have asked three or four people here [colleagues in the nursing home where she lives], and they have memories of losing people; they said 'my poor father was taken and there was no man to look after the farm, and us girls had to go and work' or something like that. My mother said that nearly every family lost somebody to the flu … I think it was that the people were worn out from the war. You could not get a drop of tea. In the last war we lived on porridge. Around where I was there was a lot of working-class people. That might be why it hit us so hard. The world was a different place then. Our aunt [whose husband died from the flu] had to go out and work, she worked on an ambulance. They used to send round an ambulance and it had to have a man and a woman on it. She had small children at the time, two girls and a boy.

Sister Wilfrid's account of her aunt having to get a job to provide for her family after the death of her husband during the pandemic raised a theme that was frequently mentioned by the interviewees, the changing economic circumstances that the flu forced on families, sometimes not only losing one or both parents but also the family home, perhaps with the children being cared for by other family members. She also introduced another theme that many of the interviewees mentioned, that there was an understanding that the disease had actually developed in the arenas of war. She said: 'I connect the flu with that war [the First World War]. The soldiers who were coming back, they would have brought it. They brought back all sorts of things.'[27]

CONCLUSIONS

The small sample cited here forms part of a collection of interviews that reveals personal insights into the effects of the disease that cannot be acquired from sources other than oral history. They provide evidence about the health, social and economic impact of the disease, how it affected individuals, families and communities in the short and long term, and how it was perceived by ordinary people rather than in the impersonal terms of newspaper records or official documents and institutional records.

These interviews represent an enduring line, a direct connection to the experience of the Spanish influenza pandemic in Ireland, and one that shows that while the flu became a history that was hidden from public view and not recorded in history books until recent years, it maintained its presence in the memories of those who lived through it and whose families suffered loss because of it. They show the human tragedies caused by the flu in a way that no other source can, telling us of the orphaned children, the widowed spouses, and the parents who lost one or more of their children in almost inexplicable circumstances, as well as the changing economic circumstances of families as a result of the death or loss of health of a breadwinner. They also document the against-the-odds survival stories, and the experiences of the children whose health was so threatened by the influenza that they were in some cases not expected to live through the night, but yet lived into their 90s like Tommy Christian, Elizabeth Molloy and R.B. McDowell. Some, like

Katie McMenamin, even lived into their 100s, out-surviving other members of the family, including those who did not catch influenza.

These, and other interviews conducted by the author, also show that using the oral history interview to tap into the experiences of influenza can be a two-way process. Not only does it provide the historian with a rich source of material not easy to access, but it provides the subject – the interviewee, who in these circumstances could be viewed as a victim – with a way to make sense of a traumatic event in their childhood that they had not been able to understand with the knowledge to hand. Through the interview process they were given information that enabled them to set their personal experience of the influenza into the context of the national and international history of the pandemic, and so, in extreme old age, they were at last able to solve this traumatic experiential puzzle of their childhood. The trauma of lost lives and altered family circumstances burdened the people interviewed for this research all their lives; for many, recalling tragic deaths proved emotionally difficult even though the event had occurred ninety years before.

For years after, the individual health of some sufferers was affected. As R.B. McDowell's interview documented, some people had to consider their career options taking into account the damage caused to their bodies by the disease. R.B. himself was left with a lifelong fascination with his own health that may well have been triggered by his early close call with death; and yet although he had been considered an invalid for most of his youth and early adulthood, he lived to extreme old age.[28] Some interviewees recalled that in later years precautions would be taken that reminded them of the time when the threat of the pandemic was present. For example, local authorities would disinfect buses when a seasonal influenza seemed to be getting particularly troublesome. Others pondered whether their parents' almost paranoid fears that they would 'catch' cold were a manifestation of post-pandemic trauma. Children were continually urged to wrap up well in layers of warm, woolly clothing, and advised not to go out with their hair wet in case they 'caught a chill'.

Unsubstantiated tales of mass burials during the influenza epidemic, particularly of children, abound.[29] The true extent of family loss in Ireland during the pandemic will never be known, but appears to be greater than the official statistics indicate.

10

'And So To Bed': Bone and Joint Tuberculosis in Children in Ireland, 1920–1950

Susan Kelly

*L*iterature concerning the history of tuberculosis has continued to expand in recent years.[1] However, this body of research has focused on pulmonary (lung) tuberculosis and mostly ignores other sites of infection, such as the bones and joints. Within the history of medicine, childhood illness has been relatively neglected. However, investigations are now beginning to open up the subject.[2] This chapter aims to place itself in this arena by exploring the experiences of children with bone and joint tuberculosis predominantly in Ireland, a country where, as Anne Mac Lellan discusses in an earlier chapter, tuberculosis was prevalent. In the opening decades of the twentieth century tuberculosis mortality was higher in both Northern Ireland and Éire than in England and Wales and Scotland.[3] The reasons for this are multi-factorial. The later emergence of a tuberculosis epidemic in Ireland, likely due to the rural nature of Irish society, may have meant that the epidemic pattern of rise, peak and fall, which usually occurred over fifty to seventy-five years, all occurred later in Ireland than in Scotland,

England and Wales. Poverty, malnutrition and overcrowding in housing all facilitated the spread of infection in the population.[4] This regional study attempts to open up the experience of children in Irish institutions between 1920 and 1950. The process of the disease was universal, but medical and nursing care, as well as institutional experiences, may have varied nationally and internationally. Further research in this area would be useful.

A combination of sources was used for this research. Oral history interviewees were found by word of mouth, visiting a daycare centre for the elderly and by placing requests in newspapers. The experiences of the interviewees relate to the decades from 1910 to 1960.[5] Personal testimonies, hospital archives, government publications and contemporary medical and nursing literature were also consulted.

This chapter asserts that sufferers of bone and joint tuberculosis, often children, were in hospital longer, were more immobilized, had a more complicated response to anti-tuberculous drugs and could be left more disfigured and with more long-term problems than their contemporaries with pulmonary tuberculosis. Official statistics often neglect the category of bone and joint tuberculosis, and even when available, such as the calculations of average time spent as an inpatient, the experience of the subgroup most badly affected is hidden in the generality of the average.

THE DISEASE: BONE AND JOINT TUBERCULOSIS

Tuberculosis is caused by *Mycobacterium tuberculosis*, that was first demonstrated by Robert Koch in 1882. This could be transmitted from person to person as human tuberculosis or from cow to person as bovine tuberculosis (caused by *Mycobacterium bovis*). The two most common routes for the bacteria to enter the body were via the stomach, if ingested, and via the lung, if inhaled. Bovine tuberculosis was most commonly transmitted via the stomach in infected milk, and human tuberculosis was most commonly transmitted when the bacillus was coughed out by one person and inhaled by another. Tuberculosis experienced by children is the same disease as that contracted by adults. The different physiology of children, however, causes it to behave differently. In adults, the *Mycobacterium* more frequently settles where it enters the body and the disease, if it becomes active, does so at this site. In children, an underdeveloped immune system means they are less able to localize infections and the disease can move about the body with greater ease. Oxygen-rich tissue is particularly vulnerable to infection. The book *Tuberculosis in Infancy and Childhood*, edited by Theophilus Nicholas Kelynack and published in 1908, included chapters on tuberculosis of children involving the nervous system, the nose and throat, the larynx (voice box), chest, abdomen, meninges (surroundings of brain), joints and spine.[6] This list delineated the variety of tuberculous conditions which doctors treated in children, and illustrated the difficulty of diagnosis. Tuberculosis can involve any structure of the body.

One of the more common secondary sites for abdominal tuberculosis, which was mostly bovine in origin, was bones or joints. This meant that many sufferers from bone and joint tuberculosis caught the disease as children from infected milk or a 'milk germ'.[7] Tuberculin testing of dairy cows and pasteurization of milk has greatly reduced this mode of transmission.[8] Bone tuberculosis could develop in any bone in the body. The common sites were the ends of the long bones (which could spread to a joint such as elbows and ankles), the hip/pelvis and the spine. A child with bone tuberculosis would complain of pain and tenderness at the site and it could appear swollen. Diagnosis was difficult and oral history interviewees often describe multiple trips to the doctor before a diagnosis was made. Some children were diagnosed only when they stopped walking due to the pain.[9] Abscesses often developed at this site. These abscesses could develop into a sinus where infected material suppurated to the surface. Spinal tuberculosis, previously known as Pott's disease, was prone to serious complications. As well as sinus formation, the collapse of an infected vertebra could lead to spinal cord compression and paraplegia. One very visible complication was kyphosis or 'hump' formation, where the kyphotic spine could compress the heart and lungs, leading to difficulty in breathing and mobility.

THE LENGTH OF STAY

Even a short stay in hospital can be traumatic for a child, but many of those who had tuberculosis, of any part of their body, had to endure very long sojourns. This was particularly the case for those who had tuberculosis of the hip or spine. In Whiteabbey Sanatorium, Belfast in 1918, the average length of stay for children with pulmonary tuberculosis was sixty-seven days, while in Throne Hospital, Belfast the average stay for children with tuberculosis of the bone and joints was 'many months'.[10] This difference was exaggerated further as the use of X-rays increased. A fully equipped X-ray apparatus, gift of the Belfast Insurance Committee in 1920, enabled medical staff to observe previously hidden changes in the bone, for better or worse, during the course of the treatment.[11] In the year March 1921 to 1922, ninety-seven X-rays were taken of the children at the Municipal Hospital for Tuberculous Children at Graymount.[12] These were felt to be very important 'since films taken at periodical intervals give a very definite indication of the process of healing … even when a sinus has been firmly healed the X-ray film may still show a good deal of rarification in the diseased bone, indicating the need for still further care and immobilization'.[13] Medically this was an advance, though it meant a longer stay for patients. By 1923 the average stay for children with bone and joint tuberculosis had extended; in Graymount Hospital it was eighteen months.[14] Table 7 shows the increasing number of X-rays taken at Graymount and then at Greenisland over the years.[15]

By 1952 the average length of stay of a child at Crawfordsburn for pulmonary tuberculosis was 161 days, while in Greenisland for bone and joint tuberculosis it was 745 days.[16] This ranged up to 1,403 days for those patients discharged in 1955.[17] Official figures for the average length of stay of patients at Greenisland were calculated by the Northern Ireland Tuberculosis Authority (NITA) for all the patients discharged each year and included the children with tuberculosis of the elbow or ankle who might be inpatients for a short length of time and also those whose sojourn ran into many years. Therefore, the average could be skewed up or down depending on the individual cases discharged that year. In Musgrave Park Hospital, Belfast the

Table 7. Annual X-Rays taken at Graymount and Greenisland

Year	Annual X-Ray Number
1923	63
1924	75
1925	25
1930	33
1932	85
1947	80
1949	95
1950	248
1953	527
1956	660

Source: Compiled from figures in Corporation of Belfast Tuberculosis Department the Report of the Chief Tuberculosis Officer (1923 –1932) and NITA Annual Reports, (1947 –1956).

average length of time spent as an inpatient for those with spinal tuberculosis was 2.25 years before chemotherapy was introduced and two years for those after chemotherapy. Sister Evelyn Pearce writing in 1939 commented, with regard to tuberculosis of the hip, that 'the period of fixation on the splint will vary with the extent of the disease, an average case probably requiring anything from eighteen months to three years'.[18] In both groups of the Musgrave Park Hospital review (pre- and post-chemotherapy) there were a number of patients who 'had become more or less permanent residents in hospital because of incurable complications'.[19] Oral history interviews show that many children with bone and joint tuberculosis of the hip or spine remained in hospital for many more years than this average.[20] Of oral history interviewees the average length of time for tuberculosis hip patients to spend in hospital was 4.25 years, while for patients with tuberculosis spine the average was six years.[21] One interviewee was an inpatient for ten years. There are records of a child who was in Greenisland with tuberculosis of the spine for fourteen years and another interviewee believed that two of his fellow patients had been resident for seventeen and eighteen years.[22]

Few parents were prepared for the lengthy stay; for some it was a slow realization, for others a rude shock on admission. One boy said his father often talked about the day he went into Downe Sanatorium, aged 4, in 1944.

> The day I was brought in, I always remember my father telling this here, my dad put my clothes in the locker and Miss M who was Matron said: 'You can take them home again, he won't be out of here for at least four years.' So it was a sickener. Oh she was quite blunt about it. They were shattered, of course.[23]

As it happened, he spent six years in Downe Sanatorium and a further two in Greenisland Hospital. There was simply no need to keep clothes in hospital for children who were going to spend years in bed and would have outgrown them by the time they were leaving.

THE TREATMENT

In 1920 Cappagh National Orthopaedic Hospital for the treatment of bone and joint tuberculosis opened near Dublin, and the following year the Municipal Hospital for Children, Graymount opened in Belfast.[24] Treatment for the condition appears at this time to have been fairly uniform throughout the British Isles with the emphasis, as in the case of pulmonary tuberculosis, on good food, fresh air and immobilization.

The site of tuberculosis in a bone or joint meant that rest was not simply bedrest, but instead immobilization of the limb or spine. On a visit to Graymount Hospital in 1922, a reporter for the *Belfast Telegraph* described the scene. In the midst of the hyperbole the three tenets of treatment can be detected. The first, fresh air and sunshine:

> Outside the house a wooden platform has been erected on which the beds are arranged in two rows, each bed occupied by a little patient. There is an awning overhead, but otherwise it is

quite open to the air. On fine days the beds are put out on the grassy lawn, quite open to the sky and blessed sunshine with all its remedial effects.[25]

Secondly, immobilization was described thus:

> ... some were strapped down, some had plaster bandages or wooden splints ... the children were happy as sand boys, notwithstanding their plaster bandages and ailments which they did not mind at all. They were every one of them, fat and rosy cheeked, bright and cheerful ... and the two little girls, Dorothy and Eileen, who smile at you 'upside down' seem to rather like it.[26]

The third tenet, good food, was described only briefly in the *Belfast Telegraph*, as 'meat, potatoes, vegetable and pudding'.[27]

These tenets of treatment remained unchanged over the decades. For example in 1939 in Cappagh Rosemary remembers that children were still watching the world inverted. '[My neighbour] had a problem with her spine ... she was put on a spinal frame which meant she was bent backwards and her head was held back. So everything she saw must have been upside-down.'[28] In 1941 the staff and children from Graymount moved to Greenisland to escape the Belfast blitz. The fresh air regime from Graymount continued, with children nursed outside as much as possible, as Jean described regarding the 1950s:

> ... each night one row of beds was put out and one row stayed inside, indoors. And then that, the next night it was the other way round ... Very, very few nights was too bad, for everybody to be inside ... even during winter. Where we slept outside there was a canopy ... you just got used to it. It was part of the routines and that was it. You just had to put up with it.[29]

Similar regimes went on in the other sanatoria. In Cappagh the children 'lay out in the open-air most of the year … summer and winter unless driving rain or snow'.[30] While in Craig-y-nos sanatorium, Wales, interviewees can remember being outside even when there was snow around. 'We were on the balcony in the snow of 1947. The nurses … put Vaseline on our faces to stop them chapping. We had green tarpaulins on the bed to keep off the rain and snow. I couldn't snuggle down because I was in this frame so I would pull the covers over my face for warmth.'[31]

While food and fresh air were considered to be curative, the main treatment was immobilization. Some of the children had tuberculosis of an upper joint but the long-stay patients had it in their spine or hip. This led to a variety of immobilization devices. Some wore a corset, which was strapped to a wooden frame on the bed, or had weights and sandbags applied to straighten limbs. According to interviewees, immobilization devices remained virtually unchanged between the 1920s and 1950s. The initial immobilization could mean a great relief from pain. One aid to diagnosis of tuberculosis of the hip was the presence of night cries.

This was due to the relaxation of the muscles controlling the joint, which during the day were constantly on guard maintaining a varying amount of rigidity; during sleep these relaxed, the sensitive areas of diseased bone rubbed together, and caused a sharp cry; the child may not have awoken, and if they did would not have been conscious of pain. A mother or nurse may have noticed that during sleep the child's hands were holding the thigh as if to support and protect it.[32]

When the weight and pulley were first fitted 'as if by magic', the pain stopped.[33] Plaster cast was the other immobilizing device, which also created problems for the children. 'Oh I'll tell you what was awful, the itch. You were in plaster from there, right down that leg … and the itch under the plaster. I can remember that as being one of the worst aspects.'[34] Children moved between these two methods of immobilization, or a combination of both, as conditions dictated:

[Staff] sealed me in a plaster cast ... from your neck to your knees. And like it was a terrible, very, very uncomfortable, very painful because then they put it on, it solidified, they had to take it off again. It stuck to the skin. So, then put it back on again. But every day, every day you had to have methylated spirits and things like that rubbed into the skin, because you got sore ... It was an awful job for the nurses because every child had to be done every day. And the stuff rubbed in to make your skin hard ... right down your back they rubbed the stuff in ... they took you out of your plaster ... unless they had the plaster sealed on. Sometimes it was sealed on ... You weren't allowed to move it off, so what they'd do was put you into a spinal jacket. They had this jacket. There would have been four straps and you'd have been strapped in with this thing. There would have been four straps on it. And they designed these ... wooden boxes we called them. They were sort of hard mattresses and a wooden box. And it was buckles in each corner and you were strapped into that. And then sometimes if it was TB in the leg they'd pack sandbags around it. They could have moved their upper part of the body, we [TB spines] couldn't move at all. So you were just lying there.[35]

Tommy describes his move from lying on his back to lying on his front.

You could see all around, you could look and see the other way ... I mean you were lying on your back for four or five or six years and then ... that experience was fantastic. And you felt a bit more normal I think, you felt a bit more alive 'cause you could contact people at eye level. Speak over to people whereas you couldn't do that before. [On your back] you couldn't hear a voice unless they actually came right over to you.[36]

ABSCESSES AND SINUSES

The treatment for abscesses and sinuses was part of the everyday life of the ward. Pus under pressure was very damaging to bone and very painful so it was important to relieve the pressure and aspirate the pus. Tommy was lucky enough not to develop an abscess or sinus but remembers seeing the others getting their dressings done: 'I used to watch the others get their treatment and I seen where theirs had opened [to the surface].'[37] Rosemary in Cappagh wasn't so lucky in this respect. She had three abscesses develop over the years she was a patient.[38]

> Another trolley, set up for the dressing of wounds, with wads of gauze and cotton wool, bottles of iodine, red mercurochrome and gentian violet. Hot sterile dressings were plucked with long tongs out of a steaming cauldron and waved about in the air until just cool enough to be placed as a hot fomentation over the affected part. Nearly every patient got a wound or two. These were caused by the bursting of abscesses which formed on the diseased limbs, swelling up the flesh ... That was bad enough, but worse by far was the treatment: the aspirating, which had to be done many times before the abscess was ready to burst open and expel the last of the poison ... the thick, hollow needle with the syringe attached was plunged into the heart of the swelling ... [and] the poison was drawn out.[39]

Cupfuls of pus were sometimes removed.[40]

> When we saw the syringe of yellow pus, we laughed with pure relief and gave thanks, for the swelling was eased and with the help of God there would be no more aspirating for a week, maybe two. In that time, the abscess might ripen and burst of its own accord ... an open wound was better than an abscess any day.[41]

For many such as Jonathan, a patient at Cappagh in the 1940s, the lasting scars remain a reminder of their abscesses and dressings.

> I was frightened of going to the operating theatre where I had many dressings changed … I also well recall my surgeon Dr M., who had a kind face and bedside manner, but I was always rather scared of him because his treatment sometimes hurt me. To this day I have a large scar on my hip where the TB drain was inserted. It had to be changed a great deal and this hurt.[42]

Sometimes patients were even sent home with them. Jack, who was in Greenisland for six years in the 1940s, remembers that the sinus on his hip remained open for a further two years after he got home.

> When I eventually got home the sinus thing was still open, was still running … My mother every day had to put a dressing on this thing. And I remember she'd a wee aluminium saucepan, she used to boil the water in it … it was a bloody nuisance because she'd put [the dressing] on and it'd be damp and maybe the sticking plaster wouldn't stick and would be hanging or twist. There would always be a slight yellowy discharge from it like a musky thing … and [after two years] the thing went away.[43]

As nurses did their daily rounds they also inspected the skin carefully for splint sores. Any red areas were dusted with powder or rubbed with methylated spirits to harden the skin. Pressure could be relieved by padding the area above and below the tender skin. Nurses were advised in the 1939 *Textbook of Orthopaedic Nursing* that:

> No complaint of discomfort should be ignored, and in the case of young children, any restlessness, fretfulness, or crying at night ought to be investigated at once. A patient old enough to

complain will probably describe pressure as a hot burning pain; this inevitably means a sore. On the other hand, the patient may not complain, and the first indication of soreness may be an offensive smell or sticky discharge.[44]

This was an unfortunate occurrence as it meant, as well as causing pain, treatment might have to be suspended and the splint removed to let the sore heal.

SURGERY

Mr Malcolm, the house surgeon at Graymount from its opening, wrote in 1933 that 'at one time there was much difference of opinion in regard to operative versus non-operative treatment. For some years conservative treatment has been regarded as the best treatment ....' In a review of the treatments used in the first ten years at Graymount (1921–31) surgery was rarely mentioned. The author stated that '... treatment is still a matter of opinion and perhaps of fashion', and he went on to describe the conservative plan of fresh air, sunshine, good food and rest of the affected area with the use of immobilizing devices. Surgery was mentioned regarding cases when 'amputation was necessary'.[45] Other surgical procedures were also performed. Mr Malcolm commented: '... it remains for the surgeon to deal with abscesses, to prevent deformities, or to correct, as far as possible, deformities that have already arisen.'[46] Neither the percentage of children who received surgery nor the frequency of these procedures was provided, so it is difficult to make direct comparisons with other hospitals.

However, the impression is given that Graymount was conservative in its use of surgery. As Mr Malcolm stated, there were two schools of opinion in orthopaedic hospitals at this time. Some hospitals may have been using a larger degree of surgical treatment. Anne Borsay describes treatment in the Royal Orthopaedic Hospital in Birmingham in 1928. A boy spent ten years there on and off and had sixteen operations over the years. Borsay makes the point that in some hospitals, parents had little choice about whether or not their children should have surgery. At the Princess Elizabeth Orthopaedic Hospital in Exeter, for example, 'withholding consent to surgical treatment not only led to boots and appliances being refused but also triggered referral to the local authority for 'such legal action ... as ... [it] may think fit to take'. It was not stated whether the orthopaedic problems of these children were caused by tuberculosis.[47] Graymount Hospital was specifically for children with bone and joint tuberculosis. Medical opinion differed in the 1920s and 1930s as to the optimum amount of surgery. However, as techniques improved, 'more frequently and more expertly applied operations' for bone and joint tuberculosis, along with antibiotics, led to a better prognosis.[48]

It is not clear from records what type of surgery was being carried out. These could range from the relatively simple aspiration of abscesses on the hip to the much more complicated and risky surgery on the spinal cord region. One boy, Harry, remembers how, some time after being discharged from Greenisland in the 1950s, he was admitted to Musgrave Park Orthopaedic Hospital for surgery.

> For what they call leg lengthening ... They cut your femur ... or fibia [sic] and put two big pins, that length ... and the nurse came along, I think it was every day, and just gave it a wee, wee slight screw, you know ... There must have been a couple of [inches growth, though] it is still three inches short.[49]

This interviewee was left with quite a limp and needed to wear a built-up shoe. This would have been even more pronounced without the leg-lengthening surgery.

THE USE OF CHEMOTHERAPY

Therapeutic drugs for the treatment of tuberculosis were developed between 1945 and 1952. They were streptomycin in 1945, para-amino salicycle acid (PAS) in 1946 and isoniazid (INAH) in 1952.[50] In many centres treatment of spinal tuberculosis remained conservative after the introduction of anti-

Table 8. Complications of Spinal Tuberculosis before and after the use of Chemotherapy

Complications	Spinal TB treated without chemotherapy	Spinal TB treated with chemotherapy
Death	10.2%	3.1%
Paraplegia	13.2%	19%
Abscess formation in adults	46.2%	42.1%
Abscess formation in children	22%	30%
Bony ankolysis (fusing)	9 years	5 years

Source: Compiled from 'Tuberculosis of the Spine: A Study of the Results of Treatment during the last Twenty-Five Years', *Journal of Bone and Joint Surgery*, 52, 4 (November 1970), pp 613-628. Study of 740 patients.

tuberculous drugs. It was hoped that chemotherapy alone would produce spectacular results, although it was realized that lesions continued to need additional drainage.[51] The introduction of anti-tuberculous chemotherapy alone could not treat active tuberculosis of the bone as an abscess had no blood supply and therefore antibiotics could not penetrate it. Surgeons found that by using early operation and adjuvant chemotherapy, a stable spine could be produced in 75 per cent of cases. This obviously left 25 per cent of patients with tuberculosis of the spine with an unstable back, and this could lead to further medical problems.

As can be seen in Table 8, chemotherapy reduced the death rate from spinal tuberculosis in this group of patients by 7.1 per cent, and bony fusion was achieved four years earlier. However, paraplegia increased by almost 5 per cent and abscess formation occurred in 8 per cent more children. It is possible that paraplegia increased after the introduction of chemotherapy as patients who would previously have died now survived but with paraplegia.

So what did this mean for individual children in Greenisland Hospital? Rachel, for example, developed tuberculosis of the spine in 1944 and spent twelve years immobilized in bed. She received five courses of streptomycin, PAS and INAH, only for an abscess to form when she was allowed up from bed.[52] Another child developed tuberculosis of the spine in 1943 at the age of 2. She spent fourteen years, between the ages of 2 and 16, immobilized. Although her strain of tuberculosis was sensitive to all three anti-tubercular drugs given, the review in 1961 states that the drugs 'made no difference'. She developed a psoas abscess, which occurs when pus from the spinal lesion tracks down to the loin region. She had this drained in 1951, 1956 and 1958. However, treatment was deemed a failure. Surgery increased the chances of a good result but it was dangerous and difficult, especially on late presentation. Skilled aftercare was necessary.

A retrospective study of spinal patients, which took place in Musgrave Park Hospital in 1961, included many patients whose disease had first been treated in Graymount or Greenisland when they were children.[53] Altogether more than a 15.2 per cent (thirty-three) of the 217 children with spinal tuberculosis, whose accounts are held in the archive, experienced some paraplegia, temporary or permanent. The vast majority were left with some kyphosis. This ranged from just a few degrees to those who were almost bent double.[54] Severe kyphosis could lead to 'pulmonary and cardiac embarrassment, backache and late onset paraplegia'.[55]

In a review of the 118 children treated at Graymount Hospital between 1921 and 1930, Mr H.P. Malcolm, the house surgeon, stated that ninety-nine (84 per cent) children were discharged as 'cured'.[56] This figure of 84 per cent has to be examined critically, however. Later standards may have been more exacting in what was considered a success, and some of the children may have had a relapse in subsequent years. This is particularly visible in an examination of the results of a retrospective Musgrave Park study of spinal patients.[57] It observed the results of treatment for spinal tuberculosis. The spreadsheet tabulated patients' results, terming them: 'failure', 'undecided', 'possible cure', 'probable cure' and 'definite cure'. Failure includes death, paraplegia, unstable spine or a marked kyphosis, with comments written into the report such as 'very deformed', 'back collapsing further', and 'spine riddled, gross kyphosis'. The description of what 'failure' means in practical terms makes sad reading. Those with paraplegia would have been bedridden until they died. Others would have led very restricted lives.

For those whose tuberculosis had been diagnosed as a child between 1900 and 1920 the failure rate was regarded as 100 per cent when figures were reviewed in 1961. This rate decreased to 67 per cent in the 1920s and 68 per cent in the 1930s. In the 1940s it dropped to 50 per cent and in 1950s to 31 per cent. Some but not all of the improvement was due to antibiotics. Mr Norman Martin, an orthopaedic surgeon at Musgrave Park in the 1960s, attributed the improvement to 'more frequently and more expertly applied operations'.[58]

DEATHS

Some patients with tuberculosis of the bone and joint died despite the treatment, both before and after the availability of the new anti-tuberculous drugs. In 1912, when mortality figures for Ireland first included deaths from bone and joint tuberculosis, forty-six children in Ireland were recorded as having died from the disease. The chronic nature of bone and joint tuberculosis meant that although the disease might have started in childhood, many deaths occurred in adulthood. The forty-six deaths of the under-15s in 1912 only made up 19.66 per cent of total deaths from bone and joint tuberculosis for all age groups.[59] Figures for a later period reveal that the only deaths from bone and joint tuberculosis in Greenisland between 1947 and 1958 occurred in 1950, 1951 and 1952 when there was one each year.[60] Throughout Northern Ireland in 1950 there were twenty deaths in all age groups from bone and joint tuberculosis, many of whom would have been suffering from the disease since childhood. By 1955 there were only three deaths in Northern Ireland from bone and joint tuberculosis, one in the 10–15 age group and the other two adults. If we examine a few time points in the 1960s we see in 1960 there were no deaths from bone and joint tuberculosis; 1962 and 1969 three adults only each year.[61] This reflects the pattern of the tuberculosis epidemic; towards the end there were fewer new cases, so deaths were among those who had established disease or who relapsed.

Patients from the 1940s, however, were very aware of deaths both at Cappagh and Greenisland, although the experience was handled quite differently. Tommy remembers that in Greenisland:

> Some of them died. I saw one of the Wilsons die. No one said it was because this happened or that, there was no explanation. They were just wheeled away, you know. And kids that you got to know like, you know. That you were [friends with them] and all of a sudden they weren't doing too good and the next thing you knew they were being wheeled away. And nobody said why.[62]

Deaths at Cappagh were treated quite differently, as Jonathan remembers regarding the 1940s:

> My recollection is that funerals were a regular occurrence in the children's ward. Certainly I can remember occasions when our beds were wheeled round into a circle and a priest would say Mass for the soul of poor little Bridget or Éamon, who had passed away to heaven in the night.[63]

Each journey to death was different – some relatively short, others long. One girl developed tuberculosis of the spine at the age of 13 in 1946, six weeks before she was hospitalized. Her illness occurred prior to the availability of anti-tuberculosis drugs. On admission she was nursed in bed for two months, then on a plaster of Paris bed for two and a half years. She died in hospital, paraplegic three years after the onset in 1949. Another boy developed spinal tuberculosis at the age of 11 in 1928. He also had tuberculosis of the kidneys, hips and bladder. He spent three and a half years in a frame at home and twenty years in an ambulatory brace. His tuberculosis, however, recurred in the 1950s and even with antibiotic treatment he became paraplegic. He remained bedridden from 1955 until his death at the age of 44 in 1961.

ETHOS OF CARE

The experience of children with bone and joint tuberculosis in Irish institutions was influenced as much by the psychological impact of being separated from their families and reliant on staff as by the physical treatment their disease dictated. Greenisland throughout the decades seems to have been a rather unhappy place for the children. It was somewhere that the children 'never had any feeling of being cared for or loved'.[64] From the 1920s onwards, oral history accounts tell of children running away or planning to do so, and of punishments, such as being put in the isolation ward for long periods, having hands tied down, sticking plaster over the mouth and threats of being put in the basement with the rats.[65] There were of course positive recollections of staff and events, but the overriding memory of most interviewees seems to be of loneliness and punishment. This was before the work of John Bowlby and James Robertson of the Tavistock Clinic, who wrote the seminal works on maternal deprivation, *Maternal Care and Mental Health* and *Young Children in Hospital*.[66] Gradually, these began to change the way hospitals were run, and throughout the 1950s the improvement was felt in many children's hospitals. However, Downe sanatorium, a small country unit, maintained a relaxed attitude throughout the 1940s. One interviewee who was moved from Downe to Greenisland experienced both regimes. In Downe, children nursed outside were able to look down the hill into the town, and nurses sat outside with the children during their lunch break. Visitors could pop in to see them as they wished, unlike the strictly regulated visiting of larger institutions such as Graymount, Greenisland, Craig-y-nos and Cappagh. The Religious Sisters of Charity ran Cappagh Hospital, with 'a strict kind of devotion'.[67] Sister Mary Finbar, who was in charge during the 1940s, is remembered as a kindly figure. 'She was like a mother to us because we weren't seeing our own mothers … we loved her.'[68] 'I so vividly remember Sister Mary's bedside prayers, her kind, smiling face, her white habit with its centrepiece of the pectoral cross and above all the warmth of her love.'[69] The altar they could see from their position on the balcony made the children feel 'protected in a heavenly way', and the religious ethos made them feel special. 'I was a chosen child … getting [my] suffering over on this earth.'[70] Ann Shaw, who was a patient in Craig-y-nos in the 1940s, comments regarding the Cappagh regime: 'Life in the Dublin Hospital … seems far less austere than in Craig-y-nos.'[71] Interviews reveal the variations between the ethos of care in the sanitoria. Institutional life, as well as the fracturing of family units and the stigma in society, led many sufferers of childhood tuberculosis to carry psychological scars into adulthood.[72]

CONCLUSIONS

Bone and joint tuberculosis is only a small part of the history of tuberculosis in general but had real and devastating consequences for those who contracted it and their families. This chapter shows that treatment for children with bone and joint tuberculosis remained virtually unchanged through the first half of the twentieth century. An observer walking into a ward in the 1940s would have seen immobilization equipment almost identical to that used for children decades earlier. Patients with bone and joint tuberculosis spent longer in hospital than their contemporaries with pulmonary tuberculosis, including a subgroup with tuberculosis of the hip or spine hospitalised for up to ten years, or indefinitely if permanent paraplegia and an unstable spine developed. Once chemotherapy in conjunction with surgery became available for early utilization, the duration of stay in hospitals decreased for many, though by no means all, patients.[73] Bone and joint tuberculosis was not simply 'cured' by chemotherapy. Nonetheless, the number of new cases gradually declined as tuberculosis became less prevalent in society. This decline resulted from the implementation of the Bacille Calmette-Guerin (BCG) vaccination, mass radiography, X-ray (particularly of schoolteachers), and an increase in bed numbers in sanatoria both for isolation and treatment. The wards gradually emptied, in many cases the beds of the tuberculous patients being taken by polio patients.

With the current rise in tuberculosis, society needs to be aware of bone and joint tuberculosis once more.[74] In the Blackburn area of England four children were diagnosed with bone and joint tuberculosis between 2006 and 2008.[75] Between 1999 and 2006 there were seventy-seven cases of bone and joint tuberculosis in children in the UK (2,643 for all age groups).[76] This highlights the importance for society, and doctors in particular, to be aware once more of tuberculosis as a possible diagnosis for bone and joint pain. Unfortunately, bone and joint tuberculosis has not been consigned to history, and the psychological and emotional effects described in this chapter will remain an issue.

NOTES

Introduction

1. We have drawn freely on the arguments of the contributors to this volume. Where references to their chapters are included, they serve as signposts to further information, rather than an exhaustive acknowledgement of their research findings.

2. See, for example, a modern study of the impact of the diagnosis, treatment and death of young cancer patients on their parents: R.L. Rohrer, 'Visiting Children with Cancer: The Parental Experience of the Children's Hospital of Pittsburg, 1995–2005', in G. Mooney and J. Reinarz (eds), *Permeable Walls: Historical Perspectives on Hospital and Asylum Visiting* (Amsterdam and New York: Rodopi, 2009), pp.131–46. For discussion of Victorian perspectives see P. Jalland, *Death in the Victorian Family* (Oxford: Oxford University Press, 1996), pp.119–42.

3. H. Cunningham, *Children and Childhood in Western Society since 1500* (Harlow: Pearson Longman, 2005), p.58.

4. G. Ashford, 'Childhood: Studies in the History of Children in Eighteenth-Century Ireland' (unpublished PhD thesis, St Patrick's College, Dublin City University, 2012), pp.90–141.

5. See, for example, H. Cunningham, 'The Employment and Unemployment of Children in England, c. 1680–1851', *Past and Present*, 126, 1 (1990), pp.5–50; C. Nardinelli, *Child Labor and the Industrial Revolution* (Bloomington and Idianapolis: Indiana University Press, 1989); H. Hendrick, 'Child Labour, Medical Capital, and the School Medical Service, c. 1890–1930', in R. Cooter (ed.), *In the Name of the Child: Health and Welfare, 1880–1940* (London and New York: Routledge, 1992), pp.45–71; L.A. Jackson, *Child Sexual Abuse in Victorian England* (London and New York: Routledge, 2002); H. Ferguson, 'Cleveland in History: The Abused Child and Child Protection, 1880–1914', in R. Cooter (ed.), *In the Name of the Child: Health and Welfare, 1880–1940* (London and New York: Routledge, 1992), pp.146–73.

6. Cunningham, *Children and Childhood*, Chapter 6.

7. Ibid. For an Irish context, see V. Crossman, 'Cribbed, Contained and Confined? The Care of Children under the Irish Poor Law, 1850–1920', *Éire-Ireland*, 44, 1 (Spring/Summer 2009), pp.37–61.

8. J. Robins, *The Lost Children: A Study of Charity Children in Ireland, 1700–1900* (Dublin: Institute of Public Administration, 1980), pp.192–3, 275–6.

9. Ibid., pp.119, 294. Philanthropic institutions were often accused of proselytizing, particularly in the case of orphans: see M. Luddy, *Women and Philanthropy in Nineteenth-Century Ireland* (Cambridge: Cambridge University Press, 1995); for Dublin specifically see M.H. Preston, *Charitable Words: Women, Philanthropy and the Language of Charity in Nineteenth-Century Dublin* (Westport and London: Praeger, 2004); for the twentieth century see O. Walsh, *Anglican Women in Dublin: Philanthropy, Politics and Education in the Early Twentieth Century* (Dublin: UCD Press, 2005).

10. See M. Luddy, 'The Early Years of the NSPCC in Ireland', *Éire-Ireland*, 44, 1 (Spring/ Summer 2009), pp.62–90; S. Buckley, 'Child Neglect, Poverty and Class: The NSPCC in Ireland, 1889–1939 – A Case Study', *Saothar: Journal of the Labour History Society*, 33 (2008), pp.57–70; see also S. Buckley, *Child Welfare, the NSPCC and the State in Ireland, 1889–1956* (Manchester: Manchester University Press, forthcoming 2013).

11. H. Marland and M. Gijswijt-Hofstra, 'Introduction', in H. Marland and M. Gijswijt-Hofstra (eds), *Cultures of Child Health in Britain and the Netherlands in the Twentieth Century* (Amsterdam and New York: Clio Medica, 2003), p.11; see A. Davin, 'Imperialism and Motherhood', *History Workshop*, 5 (Spring 1978), p.9.

12. Davin, 'Imperialism and Motherhood', p.9.

13. Marland and Gijswitj-Hofstra, 'Introduction', p.9.

14. Ibid.

15. I. Miller, *Reforming Food in Post-Famine Ireland: Medicine, Science and Improvement, 1845–1922* (Manchester: Manchester University Press, forthcoming), Chapter 7.

16. Ibid.

17. Ibid.

18. G. Jones and E. Malcolm, 'Introduction: An Anatomy of Irish Medical History', in G. Jones and E. Malcolm (eds), *Medicine, Disease and the State in Ireland, 1650–1940* (Cork: Cork University Press, 1999), p.6.

19. Luddy, 'The Early Years of the NSPCC in Ireland', pp.64–5.

20. See Anne Mac Lellan's and Laura Kelly's chapters in this volume.

21. A. Levene, 'Childhood and Adolescence', in M. Jackson (ed.), *The Oxford Handbook of the History of Medicine* (Oxford: Oxford University Press, 2011), p.321.

22. Ibid.

23. Marland and Gijswijt-Hofstra, 'Introduction', p.8.

24. Exceptions include T. Feeney, 'Church, State and Family: The Advent of Child Guidance Clinics in Independent Ireland', *Social History of Medicine (SHM)*, Advance Access 21 May 2012. While few medical historians have engaged directly with childhood illness in Ireland, several social and welfare histories have explored issues surrounding mothers

and their offspring: L. Earner-Byrne, 'Managing Motherhood: Negotiating a Maternity Service for Catholic Mothers in Dublin, 1930–1954', *SHM*, 19, 2 (2006), p.266; L. Earner-Byrne, *Mother and Child: Maternity and Child Welfare in Dublin 1922–60* (Manchester: Manchester University Press, 2007); C. Rattigan, *'What Else Could I Do?': Single Mothers and Infanticide, Ireland 1900–1950* (Dublin: Irish Academic Press, 2012); see also C. Rattigan, '"Half Mad at the Time": Unmarried Mothers and Infanticide in Ireland, 1922–1950', in C. Cox and M. Luddy (eds), *Cultures of Care in Irish Medical History, 1750–1970* (Basingstoke: Palgrave Macmillan, 2010), pp.168–90; P.M. Prior, 'Psychiatry and the Fate of Women Who Killed Infants and Young Children, 1850–1900', in Cox and Luddy (eds), *Cultures of Care in Irish Medical History*, pp.92–112; E. Farrell, *'A Most Diabolical Deed': Infanticide and Irish Society, 1850–1900* (Manchester: Manchester University Press, forthcoming 2013).

25. C. Cox and M. Luddy, 'Introduction', in Cox and Luddy (eds), *Cultures of Care in Irish Medical History*, p.5.

26. See Cunningham, *Children and Childhood*; H. Cunningham, *The Children of the Poor: Representations of Childhood since the Seventeenth Century* (Oxford: Blackwell, 1991).

27. M. Luddy and J.M. Smith, 'Editors' Introduction', *Éire-Ireland*, 44, 1 (Spring/Summer 2009), p.7.

28. Cunningham, *Children and Childhood*, p.15; Marland and Gijswijt-Hofstra, 'Introduction', p.8; R. Cooter, 'Introduction', in R. Cooter (ed.), *In the Name of the Child: Health and Welfare, 1880–1940* (London and New York: Routledge, 1992), p.2.

29. See, for example, Feeney, 'Church, State and Family'; Earner-Byrne, *Mother and Child*; M. Ó hÓgartaigh, *Kathleen Lynn: Irishwoman, Patriot, Doctor* (Dublin: Irish Academic Press, 2006).

30. Jones and Malcolm, 'Introduction', p.4.

31. G. Jones, *'Captain of all These Men of Death': The History of Tuberculosis in Nineteenth- and Twentieth-Century Ireland* (Amsterdam: Rodopi, 2001), pp.7–8.

32. See M.E. Daly, *Dublin, the Deposed Capital: A Social and Economic History, 1860–1914* (Cork: Cork University Press, 1984); J. Prunty, *Dublin Slums, 1800–1925: A Study in Urban Geography* (Dublin: Irish Academic Press, 1997); see also Conor Ward's, Ian Miller's and Laura Kelly's chapters in this volume; Jones, *'Captain of all These Men of Death'*, p.11.

33. Exceptions to this trend point to the social universality of diseases such as smallpox and the 'Spanish' influenza which transcended class.

34. C.E. Rosenberg, 'Introduction – Framing Disease: Illness, Society and History', in C.E. Rosenberg and J. Golden (eds), *Framing Disease: Studies in Cultural History* (New Brunswick, NJ: Rutgers University Press, 1992), p.xvii.

35. W.F. Bynum, *Science and the Practice of Medicine in the Nineteenth Century* (Cambridge: Cambridge University Press, 1994), p.2.

36. See for example R. Moore and S. McClean (eds), *Folk Healing and Health Care Practices in Britain and Ireland: Stethoscopes, Wands and Crystals* (New York: Berghahn Books, 2010).

37. For Ireland see J. Kelly, 'Domestic Medication and Medical Care in Late Early Modern Ireland', in J. Kelly and F. Clark (eds), *Ireland and Medicine in the Seventeenth and Eighteenth Centuries* (Farnham: Ashgate Publishing, 2010), pp.109–36.

38. R.C. Maulitz, *Morbid Appearances: The Anatomy of Pathology in the Early Nineteenth Century* (Cambridge and New York: Cambridge University Press, 1987), p.110.

39. Rosenberg, 'Introduction', p.xviii.

40. J. Kelly, 'The Emergence of Scientific and Institutional Medical Practice in Ireland, 1650–1800', in Jones and Malcolm (eds), *Medicine, Disease and the State in Ireland*, p.21; Jones and Malcolm, 'Introduction', p.1.

41. Jones, *'Captain of all These Men of Death'*, pp.10–11. For more on the significance of the Dublin Medical School see J. McGeachie, '"Normal" Development in an "Abnormal" Place: Sir William Wilde and the Irish School of Medicine', in Jones and Malcolm (eds), *Medicine, Disease and the State in Ireland*, pp.85–101.

42. Jones and Malcolm, 'Introduction', p.1.

43. W. Coleman and F.L. Holmes (eds), *The Investigative Enterprise: Experimental Physiology in Nineteenth-Century Medicine* (Berkeley, CA: University of California Press, 1988); J.E. Lesch, *Science and Medicine in France: The Emergence of Experimental Physiology, 1790–1855* (Cambridge, MA: Harvard University Press, 1984).

44. See M. Worboys, *Spreading Germs: Disease Theories and Medical Practice in Britain, 1865–1900* (Cambridge: Cambridge University Press, 2000), p.5; see also Ian Miller's chapter in this volume.

45. L.M. Geary, *Medicine and Charity in Ireland, 1718–1851* (Dublin: UCD Press, 2004), p.2.

46. Bynum, *Science and the Practice of Medicine*, p.25.

47. J. Warburton, J. Whitelaw and R. Walsh, *History of the City of Dublin, from the Earliest Accounts to the Present Time; Containing its Annals, Antiquities, Ecclesiastical History and Charters; its Present Extent, Public Buildings, Schools, Institutions Etc.; to which are added, Biographical Notices of Eminent Men and Copious Appendices of its Population, Revenue, Commerce and Literature* (London: W. Bulmer and Co., 1818), quoted in Geary, *Medicine and Charity in Ireland*, p.55.

48. Ibid.

49. A. Tanner, 'Care, Nurturance and Morality: The Role of Visitors and the Victorian London Children's Hospital', in G. Mooney and J. Reinarz (eds), *Permeable Walls:*

Historical Perspectives on Hospital and Asylum Visiting (Amsterdam and New York: Rodopi, 2009), pp.81–102.

50. The first two children's hospitals in Britain were the Hospital for Sick Children, Great Ormond Street in London (f. 1852) and the Jenny Lind Infirmary for Sick Children in Norwich (f. 1854). See Tanner, 'Care, Nurturance and Morality'; B. Lindsey, *'The Jenny': A History of the Jenny Lind Hospital for Sick Children, Norwich, 1854–2004* (Norwich: Norfolk and Norwich Hospital, 2004). For the Dublin Institution for the Diseases of Children see Conor Ward's chapter in this volume.

51. Crossman, 'Cribbed, Contained and Confined?', p.42.

52. See Ian Miller's chapter in this volume.

53. Tanner, 'Care, Nurturance and Morality', p.81.

54. See M. Finnane, *Insanity and the Insane in Post-Famine Ireland* (London: Croom Helm, 1981); C. Cox, *Negotiating Insanity in the Southeast of Ireland, 1820–1900* (Manchester: Manchester University Press, 2012).

55. See June Cooper's chapter in this volume.

56. See R.D. Cassell, *Medical Charities, Medical Politics: The Irish Dispensary System and the Poor Law, 1836–1872* (Woodbridge: Boydell, 1997); Geary, *Medicine and Charity in Ireland*; V. Crossman, *The Poor Law in Ireland, 1838–1948* (Dublin: Economic and Social History Society of Ireland, 2006); C. Cox, 'Access and Engagement: The Medical Dispensary Service in Post-Famine Ireland', in Cox and Luddy (eds), *Cultures of Care in Irish Medical History*, pp.57–78.

57. See Philomena Gorey's and Ian Miller's chapters in this volume.

58. Carsten Timmerman has made a similar point concerning the accommodation of elderly sufferers from incurable diseases in the English workhouse: C. Timmerman, 'Chronic Illness and Disease History', in Jackson (ed.), *The Oxford Handbook of the History of Medicine*, p.396–7.

59. Luddy, 'The Early Years of the NSPCC in Ireland', p.69.

60. Marland and Gijswijt-Hofstra, 'Introduction', pp.8, 24.

61. L. Pollock, *Forgotten Children: Parent–Child Relations from 1500 to 1900* (Cambridge: Cambridge University Press, 1983), pp.141–2. This argument is in contrast to that put forward by Lawrence Stone, who suggests that high child mortality rates correlated with reduced parental affection: see L. Stone, *The Family, Sex and Marriage in England, 1500–1800* (London: Weidenfeld & Nicolson, 1977), p.651–2.

62. Jalland, *Death in the Victorian Family*, pp.119, 121.

63. See Gabrielle Ashford's chapter in this volume.

64. G. Weisz, 'Regulating Specialities in France during the First Half of the Twentieth Century', *Social History of Medicine*, 15, 3 (2002), p.457.

65. For more on William Wilde, see Philomena Gorey's chapter in this volume.

66. R.T. Evanson and H. Maunsell, *A Practical Treatise on the Management and Diseases of Children*, 3rd ed. (Dublin: Fannin, 1840), p.105. For more information about this publication see Conor Ward's chapter in this volume.

67. Hannah Newton suggests that this may even have been recognized in the early-modern period: see H. Newton, '"Children's Physic": Medical Perceptions and Treatment of Sick Children in Early Modern England, c. 1580–1720', *SHM*, 23, 3 (2010), pp.456–74.

68. Anonymous, 'Fifty Years of Paediatrics', *British Medical Journal*, 2, 4738 (1951), p.1016; A.D.M. Jackson, 'A Voice for Children: The Development of British Paediatrics', *SHM*, 1, 1 (1988), pp.115–16.

69. A. Adams and D. Theodore, 'The Architecture of Children's Hospitals in Toronto and Montreal, 1875–2010', in C. Krasnick Warsh and V. Strong-Boag (eds), *Children's Health Issues in Historical Perspective* (Waterloo: Wilfrid Laurier University Press, 2005), pp.439–78.

70. These key figures are discussed in Anne Mac Lellan's and Laura Kelly's chapters in this volume.

71. W.R.F. Collis, *The State of Medicine in Ireland* (Dublin: Parkside Press, 1943), p.28.

72. F. Clarke, 'Collis, (William) Robert Fitzgerald ('Bob')', in J. McGuire and J. Quinn (eds), *Dictionary of Irish Biography* (Cambridge: Cambridge University Press, 2002).

73. Ibid.

Chapter 1

1. P. Razzell, *The Conquest of Smallpox: The Impact of Inoculation on Smallpox Mortality in Eighteenth-Century Britain* (Firlie: Caliban Books, 1977), pp.137, 183.

2. Ibid., p.136.

3. http://www.who.int/mediacentre/factsheets/smallpox/en, accessed 10 August 2009.

4. 'Lady [Caroline] Holland to Duchess of Leinster, 4 May [1768]', in B. Fitzgerald (ed.), *The Correspondence of Emily, Duchess of Leinster*, 3 vols (Dublin: Irish Manuscripts Commission, 1957), vol. i, p.535.

5. G. Ashford, 'Childhood: Studies in the History of Children in Eighteenth-Century Ireland' (unpublished PhD thesis, St Patrick's College, Dublin City University, 2012), pp.90–141. Also, on the role of women in medical care, see J. Kelly, 'Domestic Medication and Medical Care in Late Early Modern Ireland', in J. Kelly and F. Clark (eds), *Ireland and Medicine in the Seventeenth and Eighteenth Centuries* (Farnham: Ashgate Publishing, 2010), pp.109–36.

6. Ashford, 'Childhood: Studies in the History of Children in Eighteenth-Century Ireland', pp.90–141.

7. G. Smith, 'Prescribing the Rules of Health: Self-Help and Advice in the Late Eighteenth Century', in R. Porter (ed.), *Patients and Practitioners: Lay Perceptions of Medicine in Pre-Industrial Society* (Cambridge: Cambridge University Press, 2002), p.264.

8. See Kelly, 'Domestic Medication and Medical Care in Late Early Modern Ireland', pp.109–36.

9. For a perspective on the growth in the availability of patent and proprietary medicine see J. Kelly, 'Health for Sale: Mountebanks, Doctors, Printers and the Supply of Medication in Eighteenth-Century Ireland', in *Royal Irish Academy Proceedings*, 108C (2008), pp.1–38.

10. Rogers and Rutty identify notable epidemics in 1708–09, 1718, 1721, 1728–31, 1738, 1740–45, 1752 and 1766. J. Rutty, *A Chronological History of the Weather and Seasons, and of the Prevailing Diseases in Dublin with their Various Periods, Successions, and Revolutions, during the Space of Forty Years* (London: Robinson & Roberts, 1770); J. Rogers, *An Essay on Epidemic Diseases and More Particularly on the Endemial Epidemics of the City of Cork such as Fevers and Small-Pox* (Dublin: S. Powell, 1734). John Rutty (1697–1775) was a Dublin Quaker, physician and naturalist, born of Quaker parents on 25 December 1698 in Melksham, Wiltshire, England. He graduated as MD from the University of Leyden in 1723 and settled in Dublin as a physician in 1724. In London in 1770 he published *A Chronological History of the Weather and Seasons, and of the Prevailing Diseases in Dublin with their Various Periods, Successions, and Revolutions, during the Space of Forty Years*, which mentions the prevalent diseases throughout that period. He died on 27 April 1775 and was buried in a Quaker burial ground near St Stephen's Green, Dublin.

11. Rogers, *An Essay on Epidemic Diseases*, pp.91–3, 170–2.

12. Ibid., pp.108–13.

13. Rutty, *A Chronological History of the Weather and Seasons*, pp.126–7.

14. Ibid., pp.80–1.

15. Ibid., p.128.

16. Adlercron Diary, 1782–94 (National Library of Ireland (NLI), MS 4481).

17. R. Wright, 'A Further Account of Buying the Small Pox. By Mr Richard Wright, Surgeon at Haverford West', in *The Philosophical Transactions of the Royal Society of London from their Commencement in 1665 to the year 1800. Vol. 6: from 1713 to 1723* (London: Blackfriars, 1809), pp.631–2.

18. Ibid., p.630; P. Williams, 'Part of Two Letters concerning a Method of procuring the Small Pox, used in South Wales. From Perrot William, M.D. Physician at Haverford West, to Dr Samuel Brady, Physician to the Garrison at Portsmouth', *Philosophical Transactions of the Royal Society of London, 1722-23* (London, 1723), 32, pp.262–4.

19. Razzell, *The Conquest of Smallpox*, p.10.

20. E. Timoni, 'An Account of the Procuring of the Small-Pox by Incision or Inoculation; as it has for Some Time been Practised at Constantinople. Being an Extract of a Letter from Emanuel Timonius, Oxon. and Patav. M.D.S.R.S. dated Constantinople, December, 1713. Communicated by John Woodward, M.D. and S.R.S', in *The Philosophical Transactions of the Royal Society of London*, pp.88–91; J. Pylarini, 'A New and Safe Method of Communicating the Small-Pox by Inoculation, Lately Invented and Brought into Use. By Jacob Pylarini, M.D. formerly Venetian Consul at Smyrna', ibid., pp.207–10.

21. B. Robinson, *The Case of Five Children who were Inoculated in Dublin on the 26th of August 1725 by Bryan Robinson, M.D., to Which is Added the Case of Miss Rolt by one who was an Eye-Witness of it*, 3rd edn (Dublin: George Grierson, 1725).

22. S. Tissot, *Advice to People in General with Respect to their Health: Translated from the French Edition of Dr Tissot's Avis au people … Printed at Lyons; with all his Notes;… and Several Occasional Notes, Adapted to this English Translation by J. Kirkpatrick, M.D.* (Dublin: J. Hoey Senior, P. Wilson, S. Cotter, W. Sleater, J. Potts, Edinburgh, T. Becket and P. A. de Hondt, 1766), p.214; Robinson, *The Case of Five Children Who Were Inoculated in Dublin*. Samuel Auguste André David Tissot (1728–97) was a renowned eighteenth-century Swiss physician. His most famous work, published in 1761 during his lifetime, was *Avis au Peuple sur sa Santé*, arguably the greatest medical bestseller of the century.

23. A. Day (ed.), *Letters from Georgian Ireland: The Correspondence of Mary Delany, 1731–68* (Belfast: The Friar's Bush Press, 1991), 26 May 1747, p.102.

24. For example, see J. Haygarth, *An Inquiry how to Prevent the Small-Pox and Proceedings of a Society for Promoting General Inoculation at Stated Periods, and Preventing the Natural Small-Pox in Chester* (Chester: J. Monk, 1785).

25. John Ryder, Bishop of Down, Dublin, to Ryder, 12 October 1743 in A.P.W. Malcomson (ed.), *Eighteenth-Century Irish Official Papers*, vol. 2 (Belfast: Public Record Office, 1990), pp.14–15.

26. Razzell, *The Conquest of Smallpox*, pp.93–8.

27. De Latocnaye, *A Frenchman's Walk through Ireland, 1796–7 (Promenade d'un Francais dans l'Irlande)*, trans. J. Stevenson (Belfast: McCaw, Stevenson & Orr, 1917), pp.175–7.

28. W. Buchan, *Domestic Medicine: A Treatise on the Prevention and Cure of Diseases by Regimen and Simple Medicines with an Appendix containing a Dispensatory for the Use of Private Practitioners*, 3rd edn (Dublin: H. Saunders, W. Sleater, J. Potts, D. Chamberlaine, R. Moncrieffe, 1774), p.180.

29. Governors Proceedings Book, 1779–83, 16 December 1782 (NAI, BR/2006/86 (House of Industry) Box 2).

30. *Commons Journal (Ireland)*, 1797, vol. 17 (21 vols, 4/5th edn, Dublin, 1796–1800).

31. Rogers, *An Essay on Epidemic Diseases*, pp.175–80.

32. W.D. Churchill, 'The Medical Practice of the Sexed Body: Women, Men and Disease in Britain circa 1600–1740', *Social History of Medicine*, 18, 1 (2005), p.11.

33. Ibid.

34. Tissot, *Advice to the People in General*, p.233.

35. N.R. von Rosenstein, *The Diseases of Children and their Remedies*, trans. A. Sparrman (London: T. Cadell, 1776), p.72. Considered to be the founder of modern paediatrics, Nils Rosén von Rosenstein (1706–73) was a Swedish physician whose work *The Diseases of Children and their Remedies* is considered to be the first modern textbook on the subject.

36. Rogers, *An Essay on Epidemic Diseases*, p.182.

37. Buchan, *Domestic Medicine*, 3rd edn, pp.194–5.

38. T. Dimsdale, *The Present Method of Inoculating of the Small-Pox; to Which are Added, Some Experiments, Instituted with a View to Discover the Effects of a Similar Treatment in the Natural Small-Pox. With Piece by William Buchan and Baron Van Sweiten*, 7th edn (Dublin: John Exshaw, 1774), p.9. Baron Dr Thomas Dimsdale (1712–1800), holder of a medical degree from Aberdeen, Scotland, published a paper in 1767 on smallpox inoculation. In 1768 he was invited to Russia where Empress Catherine had volunteered to be inoculated against smallpox by Dimsdale as an example to her people. He practised in Hertford, England and was elected as MP for the area in 1780 and 1784.

39. Von Rosenstein, *The Diseases of Children*, p.73.

40. T.U. Sadlier (ed.), 'Diary of Anne Cooke, 1761–76', 10 January 1770, *Journal of the Kildare Archaeological Society*, 8 (1915–17), p.123.

41. Lady Louisa Conolly to Duchess of Leinster, 12 November 1786, *Leinster Correspondence*, iii, 382.

42. Noel Ross (ed.), 'The Diary of Marianne Fortescue', *Journal of the County Louth Archaeological Society*, 24 (1999), p.378.

43. The Suffolk surgeon Robert Sutton began practice as an inoculator *circa* 1757 and advertised his 'new method of inoculating for the small-pox' in the *Ipswich Journal* in May 1762. His method was popularized by his son Daniel. Razzell, *The Conquest of Smallpox*, p.9.

44. R. Houlton, *Indisputable Facts Relative to the Suttonian Art of Inoculation: with Observations on its Discovery, Progress, Encouragement, Opposition, &c. &c.* (Dublin: W. G. Jones, 1768).

45. W. Lefanu (ed.), *Betsy Sheridan's Journal: Letters from Sheridan's Sister 1784–1786 & 1788–1790* (London: Eyre & Spottiswoode, 1960), p.82.

46. Nath. Cooper to Alexander Marsden, 21 October 1796 (NAI, Official Papers 13/47).

47. R. Raughter (ed.), *The Journal of Elizabeth Bennis, 1749–1779* (Dublin: Columba Press, 2007), 8 April 1760.

48. Rogers, *An Essay on Epidemic Diseases*, pp.177–80. For a 1778 account of the process of smallpox inoculation see letters of Lady Louisa Conolly to the Duchess of Leinster, in Fitzgerald (ed.), *Leinster Correspondence*, iii, letter no. 123, 15 June 1778; letter no. 124, 18 June 1788; letter no. 125, 19 June 1778; letter no. 126, 23 June 1778; letter no. 127, 26 June 1778; letter no. 128, 28 June 1778; letter no. 136, 19 September 1778; letter no. 138, 28 September 1778.

49. Rogers, *An Essay on Epidemic Diseases*, pp.170–2.

50. Ibid., pp.170–2; Tissot, *Advice to the People in General*, pp.235–6; Buchan, *Domestic Medicine*, 3rd edn, p.181.

51. Buchan, *Domestic Medicine*, 3rd edn, p.181.

52. Razzell, *The Conquest of Smallpox*, p.31.

53. Rogers, *An Essay on Epidemic Diseases*, p.182.

54. Buchan, *Domestic Medicine*, 3rd edn, p.177.

55. Razzell, *The Conquest of Smallpox*, p.177.

56. A.W. Crosby, 'Smallpox', in K. Kiple (ed.), *Cambridge World History of Human Disease* (New York: Cambridge University Press, 1993), p.1010.

57. De Latocnaye, *A Frenchman's Walk through Ireland*, p.175.

58. John Ryder, Bishop of Down, Dublin, to Ryder, 12 October 1743, A.P.W. Malcomson (ed.), *Eighteenth-Century Irish Official Papers*, vol. ii, pp.14–15.

59. J. Kelly, 'Scientific and Institutional Practice, 1650–1800', in G. Jones and E. Malcolm (eds), *Medicine, Disease and the State in Ireland, 1650–1940* (Cork: Cork University Press, 1999), pp.30–1.

60. G. Jones and E. Malcolm, 'Introduction: An Anatomy of Irish Medical History', in Jones and Malcolm (eds), *Medicine, Disease and the State in Ireland*, p.8.

61. Lady Sarah Lennox to Duchess of Leinster, 28 November 1778, in Fitzgerald (ed.), *Leinster Correspondence*, vol. ii, 262.

62. William Drennan to Martha McTier, [nd] 1783, in J. Agnew (ed.), *The Drennan-McTier Letters*, 3 vols (Dublin: Irish Manuscript Commission, 1998–2000), vol. i, p.141.

63. De Latocnaye, *A Frenchman's Walk through Ireland*, p.175.

64. As Razzell briefly noted, and it is worthy of further exploration, natural smallpox led to the creation of focal lesions along the epididymis, resulting in male infertility.

65. A. Young, *A Tour in Ireland with General Observations on the Present State of that Kingdom made in the Years 1776, 1777 and 1778*, ed. C. Maxwell (Cambridge: Cambridge University Press, 1925), p.77.

66.	http://www.who.int/mediacentre/factsheets/smallpox/en, accessed 10 August 2009.

67.	Cited in L. Stone, *The Family, Sex & Marriage*, 1st edn (New York: Harper & Row, 1977), p.77, from O. Goldsmith, 'The Double Transformation', *Essays by Mr Goldsmith* (1765), pp.241–5.

68.	William Drennan to Martha McTier, [nd], in Agnew (ed.), *Drennan-McTier Letters*, vol. i, p.143.

69.	Although not related to smallpox, Olivia Weisser also identifies a mother's concern about potential scarring resulting from a seventeenth-century medical treatment to her daughter's face. O. Weisser, 'Reading Bumps on the Body in Early Modern England', *Social History of Medicine*, 22 (2009), p.335.

70.	William Drennan to Martha McTier, [nd], in Agnew (ed.), *Drennan-McTier letters*, vol. i, p.143.

71.	Day (ed.), *Letters from Georgian Ireland*, p.95.

72.	Lady Louisa Conolly to Duchess of Leinster, 28 September 1778, in Fitzgerald (ed.), *Leinster Correspondence*, vol. iii, p.318.

73.	J. Kelly, 'Print and the Provision of Medical Knowledge in Eighteenth-Century Ireland', in R. Gillespie and R. Foster (eds), *Irish Provincial Cultures in the Long Eighteenth Century* (Dublin: Four Courts Press, 2012), pp.33–56.

74.	Smith, 'Prescribing the Rules of Health', pp.273–5.

75.	For a fuller debate of this issue see Razzell, *The Conquest of Smallpox*.

76.	D. Brunton, 'The Problems of Implementation', in Jones and Malcolm (eds), *Medicine, Disease and the State in Ireland*, p.140.

77.	The term 'paediatric' and 'paediatrician' were not in use until the late nineteenth century, but the structures were laid in the eighteenth, and thus the use of the word was considered appropriate here.

78.	W. Bynum, *The History of Medicine: A Very Short Introduction* (Oxford: Oxford University Press, 2008), p.41.

79.	John Russell to William Wyndham Grenville, 7 July 1806, *Fortescue Mss*, vol. viii (London: Historical Manuscripts Commission, 1912), pp.223–4.

80.	Brunton, 'The Problems of Implementation', p.139.

81.	Ibid., p.140.

Chapter 2

1.	Acknowledgements: The author is indebted to Robert Mills, Librarian, and to Harriet Wheelock, Archivist, Royal College of Physicians of Ireland for their help in locating archival material and to the historians Eoin O'Brien FRCP and Richard Moore FRCGP for their advice and support.

2. *Watson's Gentleman's and Citizen's Almanack* (Dublin: Stewart & Hopes, 1826).

3. See for example M. Daly, *Dublin, the Deposed Capital: A Social and Economic History, 1860–1914* (Cork: Cork University Press, 1984); J. Prunty, *Dublin Slums, 1800–1925: A Study in Urban Geography* (Dublin: Irish Academic Press, 1997); E. O'Brien, *Conscience and Conflict: A Biography of Dominic Corrigan* (Dublin: Glendale Press, 1983).

4. O. MacDonagh, 'Ideas and Institutions, 1830–45', in W.E. Vaughan (ed.), *A New History of Ireland, vol. V: Ireland under the Union, Part I, 1801–70* (Oxford: Oxford University Press, 1989), p.193.

5. See for example M.E. Daly, *The Famine in Ireland* (Dundalk: Dundalgan Press, 1986); C. Ó Gráda, *The Great Irish Famine* (Dublin: Gill & Macmillan, 1989), pp.9–38.

6. *First Annual Report of the Registrar General, 1864* (Dublin: Her Majesty's Stationery Office, 1869).

7. T.W. Grimshaw, *Remarks on the Prevalence and Distribution of Fever in Dublin, with Appendices on Sanitary Matters in that City* (Dublin: Fannin, 1872), pp.26–8. This report was read to the Statistical and Social Society of Ireland in Dublin 2 July 1889. Courtesy of the Linen Hall Library, Belfast.

8. T.C. Speer, 'Medical Report Containing an Enquiry into the Causes and Character of the Diseases of the Lower Orders in Dublin', *Dublin Hospital Reports*, 3, 1 (1833), pp.164–200.

9. O.C. Ward, 'The Liverpool Infirmary for Children, 1851–1920', *Medical Historian*, 18 (2006–7), pp.11–20.

10. J. Rendell-Short, 'The Causes of Infantile Convulsions prior to 1900', *Journal of Paediatrics*, 47, 6 (December 1955), pp.733–9; R.A. Shanks, 'The Nature of Infantile Convulsions', *American Journal of Diseases of Children*, 78, 5 (1949), pp.764–74; M. A. Khan, S. Iqbal, F. H. Muhammad et al, 'Frequency of Hypocalcaemic afebrile Convulsions', *King Edward Medical University Annals*, 17, 1 (2011), pp.31-5.

11. D. Forsyth, *Children in Health and Disease* (London: John Murray, 1909), p.229.

12. C.M.B. Saunders, '101st Annual Meeting of the British Medical Association held in Dublin, July 1933', *British Medical Journal (BMJ)*, 2, 3788 (1933), pp.303-11.

13. H.E. Bechtel and C.A. Hoppert, 'A Study of the Seasonal Variation of Vitamin D in Normal Cow's Milk', *Journal of Nutrition*, 11, 6 (1986), pp.537–49; see also Laura Kelly's chapter in this volume.

14. E.M. Crawford, 'Dearth, Diet and Disease in Ireland, 1850: A Case Study of Nutritional Deficiency', *Medical History*, 28, 2 (1984), pp.151–61.

15. T.W. Grimshaw, *Remarks on the Prevalence and Distribution of Fever in Dublin, with Appendices on Sanitary Matters in that City* (Dublin: Fannin, 1872), pp.26–8.

16. Ibid.

17. M. Craft, 'The Development of Dublin: Background to the Housing Problem', *Studies*, 59, 235 (1970), pp.301–13.

18. F.O.C. Meenan, 'Victorian Doctors in Dublin', *Irish Journal of Medical Science* (*IJMS*), 1, 7 (1968), pp.311–20.

19. D.A. Coakley, *A Pride of Professors* (Dublin: A. & A. Farmar, 1999), pp.82–3.

20. In 1804, the Walkerite Sect, which espoused an extreme form of Calvinism, was founded by John Walker, a fellow of Trinity College Dublin and a former Church of Ireland minister.

21. J. Crampton, 'Case of an Anomalous State of the Heart', *Transactions of the Association of Fellows and Licentiates of the King's and Queen's College of Physicians in Ireland*, 1 (1830), pp.134–40.

22. J. Crampton, 'Cyanosis', *The Cyclopaedia of Practical Medicine*, 1 (London: Sherwood, Gilbert & Piper, 1832), pp.500–1.

23. R.C. Bentley Todd, *Cyclopedia of Anatomy and Physiology*, 2 (London: Longman Brown, 1831), p.634.

24. T. Peacock, *Malformation of the Human Heart: With Original Cases* (London: John Churchill, 1858), p.30.

25. J.A. Stewart, *A Practical Treatise on the Diseases of Children*, 3rd edn (New York: Harper, 1845), p.19.

26. E. Bedford, 'An Account of Aortic Incompetence by Thomas Cuming (1798–1887)', *Medical History*, 11, 4 (1967), pp.398–401.

27. T. Cuming, 'A Case of Cancrum Oris', *Dublin Hospital Reports*, 4 (1827), p.537.

28. T. Holes, *Surgical Treatment of the Diseases of Infancy and Childhood* (London: Robson & Sons, 1869), p.360; C. Elliotson, 'Presidential Address', *Lancet*, 19, 475 (1832–33), p.59.

29. O.C. Ward, 'The Royal College of Surgeons 19th-Century Textbook of Paediatrics and its Authors Maunsell and Evanson', *Journal of the Irish Colleges of Physicians and Surgeons*, 31, 2 (2002), pp.101–4.

30. 'Review', *Edinburgh Medical and Surgical Journal*, 51 (1839), pp.166–88.

31. R. Blayney, 'Henry Maunsell (1806–79): An Early Community Physician', *IJMS*, 153, 1 (1984), pp.42–3.

32. R.T. Evanson, 'Report on a Case in Which a Foreign Body was Supposed to be Present in the Trachea', *Dublin Journal of Medical and Chemical Science* (*DJMCS*), 5, 13 (1834), pp.19–20.

33. Hansard, 1843; 413XInf 64–9.

34. Ibid.

35. See the leading article, 'The Smyly Testimonial', *BMJ*, 1, 211 (1865), p.42.

36. Ibid.

37. D. Cheyne, *Essays on the Diseases of Children with Cases and Dissections* (Edinburgh: Maunsell, Day & Stephenson, 1801), p.1.

38. W. Stokes, 'Observations on the Treatment of Various Diseases', *DJMCS*, 1 (1822), pp.145–56.

39. D. Corrigan, 'Pica or Dirt Eating in Children', *Dublin Hospital Gazette*, 6, 13 (1859), pp.10–13.

40. D. Corrigan, 'Treatment of Incontinence in Youth by Collodion', *Dublin Quarterly Journal of Medical Science*, 49 (1870), pp.113–16.

41. D. Coakley, *Baggot Street: A Short History of the Royal City of Dublin Hospital* (Dublin: Governors of Royal City of Dublin Hospital, 1995).

42. L. Symes, 'On the Mortality of Children in Ireland 1886–1896', *DJMS*, 105 (1898), pp.479–86.

43. R. Moore, *Leeches to Lasers* (Killala: Morrigan, 2002), p.238.

44. J.W. Moore, 'Some Recent Clinical Records', *IJMS*, 5, 10 (1923), pp.507–14.

45. J.W. Moore, 'The Treatment of Children', *IJMS*, 6, 12 (1926), pp.671–82.

46. J.W. Moore 'Chronicle', *IJMS*, 6, 82 (1932), pp.616–18.

47. H. Fleetwood Churchill and G. Fleetwood Churchill, *The Diseases of Children* (Dublin: Fannin, 1858).

48. 'Review', *Lancet*, 71, 1799 (1858), p.192.

49. 'Obituary, Fleetwood Churchill', *BMJ*, 1, 894 (1878), pp.247–8.

50. 'Obituary, Charles West', *BMJ*, 1, 1944 (1898), pp.921–3.

51. C. West, *Lectures on the Diseases of Infancy and Childhood* (London: Longman, 1848).

52. Ibid.

53. H. Kennedy, *Some Account of the Epidemic of Scarlet Fever which Prevailed in Dublin from 1834 to 1843* (Dublin: Fannin, 1843).

54. R. Steen, 'Hurler's Polydystrophy with Cardiac Lesions', *British Heart Journal*, 21, 2 (1958), pp.269–74; W.R.F. Collis, 'Acute Rheumatism and Haemolytic Streptococci', *Lancet*, 27, 5625 (1931), pp.1341–5; E. Doyle, 'Coming of Age', *Journal of the Irish Medical Association (JIMA)*, 72, 1 (1979), pp.6–13; N.V. O'Donohoe, *Epilepsies of Childhood*, 2nd edn (London: Butterworth & Co., 1985); H. Hoey and M. O'Leary, 'The National Children's Hospital', in D. Fitzpatrick, *The Feds: An Account of the Federated Dublin Voluntary Hospitals 1961-2005* (Dublin: A & A Farmar, 2006), pp.42-5. I. Temperley, 'The Treatment of Coagulation Factor Deficiencies', *JIMA*, 66, 2 (1973), pp.42–5.

Chapter 3

1. There is currently no published study of the history of this hospital or its patients. Among those who have studied the Westmoreland Lock Hospital (WLH) and its

patients are Maria Luddy, who discusses the WLH and some of its patients as part of her study: M. Luddy, *Prostitution and Irish Society, 1800-1940* (Cambridge and New York: Cambridge University Press, 2007); G. Boyd, *Dublin 1745-1922: Hospitals, Spectacle and Vice* (Dublin: Four Courts Press, 2006); J. Walker, 'Westmoreland Lock Hospital, Dublin, and the Treatment of Syphilis' (unpublished PhD Thesis, NUI Maynooth, 2010).

2. John Morgan (1829–76), born in Dublin, the nephew of Arthur Jacob, was a surgeon at Dublin's Mercer hospital, WLH and Professor of Anatomy at the Royal College of Surgeons in Ireland. He was the author of a number of books and articles on sexually transmitted diseases. See C.A. Cameron, *History of the Royal College of Surgeons in Ireland, and of the Irish Schools of Medicine* (Dublin: Fannin & Co., 1886); Obituaries (Kirkpatrick Collection, Royal College of Physicians of Ireland (RCPI), Kildare Street, Dublin).

3. Westmoreland Lock Hospital Archive, RCPI.

4. 1868 is the year prior to the opening of government lock hospitals in Kildare and Cork, and a speculative possibility is that a different form of register was kept in this period with the register remaining as the property of the government. From 1869 until 1882 WLH was in receipt of a grant from the War Office and subject to inspection. The minute books of the board of governors meetings are not available for the mid-nineteenth century either. The legend of the WLH collection is that after the closure of the hospital the volumes were being incinerated until what remained were salvaged by Professor Kirkpatrick who presented them to the RCPI (with thanks to RCPI archivist Mr Robert Mills for this information).

5. A. Colles, *Practical Observations on the Venereal Disease, and on the Use of Mercury* (Dublin: Fannin & Co., 1837).

6. Sir Philip Crampton (1777–1858) was known as 'flourishing Phil' on account of his high society lifestyle and flamboyant dress. He dined regularly at the vice-regal lodge and was an accomplished musician. As a founder of the Meath Hospital and a hospital for children in Pitt Street, Dublin he was professionally ambitious and successful. Crampton became a major figure in the development of public health policies in Ireland. T. Farmar, *Patients, Potions and Physicians: A Social History of Medicine in Ireland, 1654–2004* (Dublin: A. & A. Farmar, 2004), pp.69–70; D. Coakley, *Irish Masters of Medicine* (Dublin: Town House Press, 1992), p.101; see also Conor Ward's chapter in this volume.

7. Carmichael drew greatly on his experience of venereal diseases treated at the WLH for his medical textbooks. His favoured treatments included sarsaparilla, lancing, venesection and, when all else failed, mercurial treatments. R. Carmichael, *An Essay on Venereal Diseases and the Uses and Abuses of Mercury in Their Treatment*, 2nd edn (London: Longman, 1825).

8. P. Diday, *A Treatise on Syphilis in Newborn Children and Infants at the Breast* (London: New Sydenham Society, 1859). Each of the doctors mentioned were associated with the WLH.

9. When speaking contemporaneously, the term 'venereal disease' will be used; otherwise modern terms will be used.

10. *Report of the Committee Appointed to Enquire into the Pathology and Treatment of Venereal Disease with the view to Diminish the Injurious Effects on the Men of the Army and Navy, with Appendices, and the Evidence Taken Before the Committee*, BPP, 1867–8 (4031) xxxvii.425 (Skey Committee, hereafter); *Minutes of Evidence Given before the Select Committee on the Contagious Diseases Act (1866) Report, Proceedings, Minutes of Evidence, Appendix*, Index BPP, 1868–9 (306), vii; *Report of the Select Committee on the Administration and Operation of the Contagious Diseases Acts of 1866–69*, BPP, 1880 (114), viii. 283; *Report of the Select Committee on the Administration and Operation of the Contagious Diseases Acts 1866–69*, BPP, 1881 (351), viii. 193; *Report of the Select Committee on the Administration and Operation of the Contagious Diseases Acts 1866–69*, BPP, 1882 (340), ix. 1.

11. Admiral Sir William F. Martin, before the Skey Committee, 24 November, 1865, p.565, Q. 6982.

12. Ibid.

13. These acts are extensively discussed by J. Walkowitz, *Prostitution and Victorian Society: Women, Class, and the State* (Cambridge: Cambridge University Press, 1980); M. Spongberg, *Feminizing Venereal Disease: The Body of the Prostitute in Nineteenth-Century Medical Discourse* (New York: New York University Press, 1997); M. Luddy 'An Outcast Community: The Wrens of the Curragh', *Women's History Review*, 1, 3 (1992), pp.341–55. E. Malcolm, '"Troops of Largely Diseased Women": VD, the Contagious Diseases Acts and Moral Policing in Nineteenth-Century Ireland', *Irish Economic and Social History*, 26 (1999), pp.1–14.

14. Babies born to syphilitic mothers might not always display signs of congenital infection at birth, and it is now known that they sometimes test negative for the *Treponema Pallidum* spirochaete for a period of time after birth, but that they can develop signs within days or weeks.

15. *Jam Fatalem Typum Insculpsit Senectus Maxime Praecox*; Diday, *A Treatise on Syphilis in Newborn Children and Infants at the Breast*, p.85. Diday attributed this phrase to the eighteenth-century doctor Faguer.

16. Examples include K. Holmes, P. Sparling, P. Mardh, S. Lemon, W. Stamm, P. Piot, J. Wasserheit (eds), *Sexually Transmitted Disease*, 2nd edn (New York: McGraw-Hill, 2001).

17.	J.D. Randolf, P.J. Sanchez, K.F. Schulz and F.K. Murphy, 'Congenital Syphilis', in Holmes et al., *Sexually Transmitted Diseases*, p.1165. Interstitial keratitis is the term used to describe a chronic infection of the cornea and is primarily associated with syphilitic infection. Jonathan Hutchinson was a distinguished doctor specializing in sexually transmitted diseases and writing from the 1850s to the 1870s.

18.	Associated with an infant with florid syphilis. With thanks to Professor Conor Ward for this information, supplied at the Paediatrics Workshop on 10 December 2010.

19.	The syphilitic condition known as general paralysis of the insane was not recognized by Fournier until 1870 and is associated with the latter stages of syphilis. In junior cases it would rarely manifest itself before the ages of 9 to 16 and was never listed as one of the diseases treated at the WLH before 1900. Gayle Davis noted that of the 910 neuro-syphilitic patients she sampled among four Scottish psychiatric institutions, only seven junior cases of general paralysis of the insane were recorded, all in the Barony Parochial Institution. G. Davis, *'The Cruel Madness of Love': Sex, Syphilis and Psychiatry in Scotland, 1880–1930* (Amsterdam and New York: Rodopi, 2008), p.32.

20.	J. Morgan, *Practical Lessons in the Nature and Treatment of Affections Produced by the Contagious Diseases* (Philadelphia: Lippincott, 1872), p.301.

21.	R. Evanson and H. Maunsell, *A Practical Treatise on the Management and Diseases of Children*, 5th edn (Dublin: Fannin, 1846), p.352.

22.	St John's Fever and Lock Hospital, Limerick was founded by Lady Hartstonge in the mid-eighteenth century and treated venereal cases until 1849, when an increase in cases of fever forced their exclusion. Admissions of all patients were by recommendation of a board member and subject to the board's approval. Admissions were restricted to residents of particular Limerick parishes unless they were exceptional cases.

23.	'We never refuse a woman admittance; we have no power to do so,' stated Dr Robert Shekleton, master of the Rotunda Lying-In Hospital in evidence to the *Report from the Select Committee on Dublin Hospitals*, 1854 (338), p.41, q.614; 'Being in the condition requiring medical attendance is the passport of admission,' said Mr Hugh Leonard, registrar of the Coombe hospital, in evidence to the *Commission of Enquiry into the Management and Working of Hospitals in the City of Dublin*, 1887 [C. 5042], p.112, q.2557.

24.	Cited in C. Ó Gráda, 'Dublin's Demography in the Early Nineteenth Century', *Population Studies*, 45, 1 (1991), pp.43–54.

25.	W. Thompson, figures submitted to the *Royal Commission on Venereal Disease, 1916* [CD 8189], Appendix III, Table 3, p.83.

26.	Catherine Waters, admitted 27 November 1863, General Register of Patients 1857–68, WLH Archive.

27. 3 June 1864, General Register of Patients 1857–68, WLH Archive.

28. Rosanna Courtney, admitted 19 August 1864, General Register of Patients 1857–68, WLH Archive.

29. Ibid.; Ellen MacAuley, admitted 12 July 1864.

30. J. Morgan, 'Clinical Review of Cases under Treatment at the Westmoreland Lock Hospital during the Past Six Months', *Dublin Quarterly Journal of Medical Science* (*DQJMS*), 48, 2 (November 1869), pp.506-28.

31. In the nosological table appended to J.M. Neligan, *Medicines: Their Uses and Modes of Administration*, 6th edn, ed. R. MacNamara (Dublin: Fannin, 1864), p.731ff, MacNamara, who was later a surgeon at the WLH, gave recommendation for dosages appropriate to children and indicated those unsuitable for infants.

32. Morgan, *Practical Lessons in the Nature and Treatment of Affections Produced by the Contagious Diseases*, p.307. It is probable that this practice was more likely to be used when treating children privately rather than in the WLH; however, evidence that making medicines palatable for children was a longstanding tradition is presented by H. Newton, 'Medical Perceptions and Treatment of Sick Children in Early Modern England, 1589–1720', *Social History of Medicine*, 23, 3 (2010), pp.456–74.

33. Evidence given before the Skey Committee, p.487. Thomas Byrne, MB, MRCSI was a surgeon to the Westmoreland Lock Hospital, Dublin from 1833 until 1869. F. Churchill, *On Diseases of Children* (Philadelphia: Lea & Blanchard, 1856) discusses the syphilitic condition in children at length in his text (p.705ff). He endorses the use of Brodie's stocking among other remedies (p.719ff).

34. Morgan, *Practical Lessons in the Nature and Treatment of Affections Produced by the Contagious Diseases*, p.285.

35. Among its many side effects, mercury had a purgative effect on the body when administered internally and would affect the skin when applied topically. For a discussion on the effects of mercury on children, see Churchill, *On Diseases of Children*, p.719.

36. Thomas Byrne, *Evidence given before Select Committee on Dublin Hospitals*, 1854 (338), p.4, q.39.

37. T. Byrne evidence given before the Skey Committee, p.487.

38. In children the inability to ingest nourishment contributed to their rapid decline. Morgan, *Practical Lessons in the Nature and Treatment of Affections Produced by the Contagious Diseases*, p.176.

39. Last Will and Testament of Thomas Byrne, AB, MB, FRCSI (NAI, Dublin, file T7344).

40. Morgan, 'Clinical Review of Cases under Treatment at the Westmoreland Lock Hospital during the Past Six Months', pp.506–28.

41. J. Morgan, 'A New View on the Propagation and Treatment of Venereal Disease: Successful Treatment by Inoculation Derived from a Hitherto Unknown Source with Illustrative Cases', *Dublin Journal of Medical Science*, 50, 99 (August 1870), pp.49–93, at p.58.

42. Ibid., p.58.

43. Ibid., p.60.

44. It has been observed by Albert R. Jonsen that the debate on medical that which began in the 1840s in America happened much later in Britain, where the medical profession was longer established and the integrity and clinical judgement of practitioners was relied upon. A.R. Jonsen, *A Short History of Medical Ethics* (Oxford and New York: Oxford University Press, 2000), p.62. While Morgan professionally corresponded with the surgeon at the Cork and Kildare CDA Lock Hospitals, he considered that the Dublin hospital should remain a voluntary one. Morgan, *Practical Lessons in the Nature and Treatment of Affections Produced by the Contagious Diseases*, pp.334–5.

45. WLH board room resolution, 30 September 1870, proposed by Alderman Mackey and seconded by Alderman Campbell. A copy is included with a letter from John Morgan to CSO, 19 October 1870 (NAI, CSO, RP, box 2049/1870, file 19188).

46. NAI, CSO, RP, box 2049/1870, file 19188.

47. Morgan's interrupted experiments with inoculation anticipated those carried out later by Dr Ducrey in France, who, like Morgan, inoculated the skin of patients with toxic material from infected ulcers. At weekly intervals Ducrey inoculated a new site with material from the most recent ulcer and was able to maintain serial ulcers through fifteen generations. In 1892 the bacillus he isolated was named after him, *Bacillus Ducreii*. See A.R. Ronald and W. Albritton, 'Chancroid and Haemophilus', in Holmes et al. (eds), *Sexually Transmitted Diseases*, p.515.

48. Letter from John Morgan to CSO, 19 October 1870 (NAI, CSO, RP, box 2049/1870, file 19188).

49. Particularly in the controversial 'Oslo Study' instigated twenty years later by Caesar Boeck, which traced the course of syphilis in untreated patients and which was followed up in 1949 and 1951 yielding valuable yet ethically questionable information to students of the disease. In order to observe the natural progression of the disease, participants in the study were given no treatment. See P. Sparling, 'Natural History of Syphilis', in Holmes et al. (eds), *Sexually Transmitted Diseases*, p.473ff.

50. Morgan, *Practical Lessons in the Nature and Treatment of the Affections produced by the Contagious Diseases*, p.297.

51. Ibid., p.311. Both Diday in *Infantile Syphilis* (1859) and Morgan in *Practical Lessons in the Nature and Treatment of Affections Produced by the Contagious Diseases* raise this issue.

52. J. Harsin 'Syphilis, Wives and Physicians: Medical Ethics and the Family in Late Nineteenth-Century France', *French Historical Studies*, 16, 1 (1989), pp.72–95.

53. Morgan, *Practical Lessons in the Nature and Treatment of Affections Produced by the Contagious Diseases*, p.311.

54. Ibid., p.93; also Morgan, 'Cases Under Treatment at the Westmoreland Lock Hospital', p.515.

55. The husband would not have been treated at the hospital but could have been treated as an outpatient at any of the city dispensaries, or as an inpatient at Dr Steevens' hospital.

56. William Wilde earned wide support from his Dublin medical colleagues in his defence of Amos Greenwood in England, who was tried and convicted for the murder of a child whom he was alleged to have raped and infected with syphilis and who subsequently died. Morgan, *Practical Lessons in the Nature and Treatment of Affections Produced by the Contagious Diseases*, p.309; W.R. Wilde, *Medico-Legal Observations Upon Infantile Leucorrhoea* (Dublin: Fannin, 1853); J.B. Lyons, 'Sir William Wilde's Medico-Legal Observations', *Medical History*, 41, 4 (1997), pp.437–54.

57. Morgan, 'Clinical Review of Cases under Treatment at the Westmoreland Lock Hospital', p.514.

58. Until 1883 no written guidelines were published by the General Medical Council on the regulation of professional conduct, although cases were heard from 1861. R.G. Smith, 'The Development of Ethical Guidance for Medical Practitioners by the General Medical Council', *Medical History*, 37, 1 (1993), pp.56–67.

59. M. Spongberg discusses this in 'Written on the Body: Degeneracy, Atavism and Congenital Syphilis: Re-reading Child Prostitution in the Nineteenth Century', *Journal of Interdisciplinary Gender Studies*, 1, 1 (1995), pp.8–88.

60. Morgan, *Practical Lessons in the Nature and Treatment of Affections Produced by the Contagious Diseases*, p.71.

61. Ibid., p.298.

62. D. McLoughlin, 'Women and Sexuality in Nineteenth-Century Ireland', *Irish Journal of Psychology*, 15, 2–3 (1994), p.270.

63. Spongberg, *Feminizing Venereal Disease*.

64. This case was in the Richmond Hospital and was discussed at length by Thomas Byrne at the 1854 commission into the operation of Dublin hospitals.

65. *Board of Superintendence, 31st Annual Report*, p.5.

Chapter 4

1. W. Mackenzie, *A Practical Treatise on the Diseases of the Eye* (London: Longman, Rees, Orme, Brown & Green, 1830), pp.334–6; A. Jacob, 'On Diseases of the Eye as a Guide in the Study of Pathology', *Dublin Medical Press*, 13 April 1842, p.225.

2. Mackenzie, *A Practical Treatise*, 4th edn, 1854, p.454; W. Lawrence, *A Treatise on the Diseases of the Eye* (Philadelphia: Lea & Blanchard, 1854), pp.254, 256; H.W. Williams, *A Practical Guide to the Study of the Diseases of the Eye: Their Medical and Surgical Treatments* (Boston: Ticnor & Fields, 1862), pp.45–7; H.C. Angell, *A Treatise on Diseases of the Eye* (Boston: James Campbell, 1870), pp.85–6.

3. For examples of overcrowding see L.M. Geary, *Medicine and Charity in Ireland, 1718–1851* (Dublin: UCD Press, 2004), pp.185–8.

4. [2] *Fourth Annual Report of the Commissioners for Administering the Laws for Relief of the Poor in Ireland: with Appendices, Ophthalmic Diseases in Workhouses: Reports from Medical Practitioners, Appendix A, No. IX*, BPP 1851 (1381), xxxvi, p.8.

5. F. Kirkpatrick, 'The Epidemic Ophthalmia of the Irish Workhouses', *Dublin Quarterly Journal of Medical Science* (May 1856), p.5.

6. *The Census of Ireland for the Year 1851, Part IV, Report on Ages and Education; Report on Tables of Deaths*, BPP 1856 (2053), lviii, p.313.

7. W. Wilde, 'On the Epidemic Ophthalmia which has Prevailed in the Workhouses and Schools of the Tipperary and Athlone Unions', *London Journal of Medicine*, 3, 25 (January 1851), p.19.

8. *Kanturk Union. Statement of the number of persons who have become blind, or who have lost the sight of one eye, in the workhouses of the Kanturk Union, during the present and past year; also, copies of medical reports made by order of the Poor Law Commissioners on the prevalence of eye diseases in these workhouses; and dates and extracts of copies of reports made to the commissioners by Poor Law inspectors, calling their attention to this subject, and resolutions of boards of guardians*, BPP 1852 (265), xlvi, p.2.

9. H.C.G. Matthew and B. Harrison (eds), *Oxford Dictionary of National Biography* (Oxford: Oxford University Press, 2004).

10. A. Jacob, 'An Account of a Membrane in the Eye, Now First Described', in *Abstracts of Papers Printed in the Philosophical Transactions of the Royal Society of London*, vol. II, 1815–1830 (London: Royal Society of London,1833), pp.116–17.

11. See Conor Ward's chapter in this volume for more information on Maunsell.

12. T.G. Wilson, *Victorian Doctor: Being the Life of Sir William Wilde* (New York: L.B. Fischer, 1846), pp.88–95.

13. Ibid., pp.47–51.

14. Ibid., pp.96–104.

15. J. McGeachie, '"Normal" Development in an "Abnormal" Place: Sir William Wilde and the Irish School of Medicine', in E. Malcolm and G. Jones (eds), *Medicine, Disease and the State in Ireland, 1650–1940* (Cork: Cork University Press, 1999), pp.85–101.

16. P. Froggatt, 'Sir William Wilde, 1815–1876: Demographer and Irish Medical Historian', in Eiléan Ní Chuilleanáin (ed.), *The Wilde Legacy* (Dublin: Four Courts Press, 2003), pp.51–68; 'Sir William Wilde and the 1851 Census of Ireland', *Medical History*, 9, 4 (October 1965), pp.302–27.

17. *Medical Directory for Ireland 1852. Supplemental list.*

18. *Fourth Annual Report, Appendix A*, no. IX, p.135.

19. An Act for the more Effectual Relief of the Destitute Poor in Ireland, 31 July 1838 (1&2 Vic., c.56); C. Kinealy, *This Great Calamity: The Irish Famine, 1845–52* (Dublin: Gill & Macmillan, 2006), pp.22–6; L.M. Geary, *Medicine and Charity in Ireland, 1718–1851* (Dublin: UCD Press, 2004), p.158; V. Crossman, *The Poor Law in Ireland, 1838–1948* (Dundalk: Dundalgan Press, 2006), p.8.

20. *Fourth Annual Report, Ophthalmic Diseases in Workhouses*, p.8.

21. *Fifth Annual Report of the Commissioners for Administering the Laws for Relief of the Poor in Ireland: with Appendices. Appendix B*, no. XVI, Summary of Returns of the Numbers of Cases of Ophthalmia, BPP 1852 (1530), xxiii, p.208.

22. *Fourth Annual Report, Ophthalmic Diseases in Workhouses, Reports from Medical Practitioners, Appendix A*, no. IX, p.136.

23. Williams, *A Practical Guide to the Study of the Diseases of the Eye*, p.45.

24. Kirkpatrick, 'The Epidemic Ophthalmia of the Irish Workhouses', p.7.

25. Ibid., p.8.

26. E.M. Crawford, 'Dearth, Diet and Disease in Ireland, 1850: A Case Study of Nutritional Deficiency', *Medical History*, 28, 2 (1984), p.151.

27. For a discussion on the growth of dependence on the potato in the pre-Famine period see D. Dickson, 'The Potato and Irish Diet before the Famine', in C. Ó Gráda (ed.), *Famine 150: Commemorative Lecture Series* (Dublin: Teagasc/University College Dublin, 1997), pp.1–27; M.E. Daly, 'Farming and the Famine', in ibid. pp.29–48; M.E. Daly, *The Famine in Ireland* (Dundalk: Dundalgan Press, 1986), pp.1–51; C. Ó Gráda, *The Great Irish Famine* (Dublin: Gill & Macmillan, 1989), pp.9–38.

28. G. Phillips, *The Potato Disease: Its Origin, Nature and Prevention* (London: S. Highley, 1845); I. Miller, 'The Chemistry of Famine: Nutritional Controversies and the Irish Famine c. 1845–7', *Medical History*, 56, 4 (October 2012), pp.444-62.

29. Crawford, 'Dearth, Diet and Disease in Ireland', p.152. It is worth noting that there was no knowledge of vitamins at the time.

30. Ibid. p.153; see also L.A. Clarkson and E.M. Crawford, 'Dietary Directions: A Topographical Survey of Irish Diet, 1836', in R. Mitchison and P. Roebuck (eds), *Economy and Society in Scotland and Ireland, 1500–1939* (Edinburgh: John Donald Publishers Ltd., 1988), pp.171–92.

31. *Kilrush and Ennistymon Unions. Return to an Order of the Honourable the House of Commons, dated 11 April 1851; – for Return "of the Deaths in the Kilrush and Ennistymon Workhouses, Hospitals, Infirmaries, and Auxiliaries, from the 25*th *Day of March 1850 until the 25*th *Day of March 1851, with the Name, Age, Sex, Causes of Death, Date of Death, Date of Admission, with the Observation of Medical Officer on each case"; "Copy of the Dietary ordered or sanctioned by the Commissioners of Poor Laws, for all classes in the Kilrush and Ennistymon Workhouses during the above period, specifying the kind of Food uses, and showing what deviation there may have been (and under what authority) from such prescribed dietary within the same period, particularly as regards the diminution of milk"; "Copy of any Correspondence between the Commissioners of Poor Laws, their inspectors, and the guardians of the Kilrush and Ennistymon Unions, with reference to the Mortality occurring within the Respective Workhouses, and of their General Management, within the 25*th *Day of March 1850 and the 25*th *Day of March 1851"; "and, Return of the Name, Rank, Salary, and Duty of each Officer and Servant at present employed in the Workhouses of Kilrush and Ennistymon"*, BPP 1851 (484), xlix, p.47.

32. *Seventh Annual Report of the Poor Law Commissioners, with Appendices, Appendix C*, BPP 1841, Session 1 (327), xi, p.157.

33. *Eighth Annual Report of the Poor Law Commissioners, with Appendices*, BPP 1842 (389), xix, p.32.

34. *Twelfth Annual Report of the Poor Law Commissioners, with Appendices*, BPP 1846 (704), xix, p.25.

35. See many examples of the difficulties experienced by local guardians as funds became depleted in *Copies of Extracts of Correspondence Relating to the State of Union Workhouses in Ireland*, BPP 1847 (766) (790) (863), lv.

36. *Kilrush and Ennistymon Unions. Return to an Order of the Honourable the House of Commons, dated 11 April 1851*, BPP 1851 (484), pp.51, 80.

37. Wilde, 'On the Epidemic Ophthalmia', p.21.

38. *Fourth Annual Report, Ophthalmic Diseases in Workhouses, Reports from Medical Practitioners, Appendix A*, no. IX, p.137.

39. Wilde, 'On the Epidemic Ophthalmia' *London Journal of Medicine*, p.23.

40. Ibid., p.23.

41. J.S. Wells, *A Treatise of the Diseases of the Eye*, 2nd edn (Philadelphia: Henry C. Lea, 1873), p.17.

42. *Fourth Annual Report, Ophthalmic Disease in Workhouses, Reports from Medical Practitioners, Appendix A*, no. IX, p.148.

43. *Fourth Annual Report, Ophthalmic Disease in Workhouses, Reports from Medical Practitioners, Appendix A*, no. IX, Copy of letter from W.R. Wilde to the medical

attendants of the workhouse of Tipperary Union, on Ophthalmic disease therein, iii, pp.144–6.

44. Wilde, 'On the Epidemic Ophthalmia', p.39.

45. *Fourth Annual Report, Appendix A, No. IX, Circulars, No. 24, Ophthalmic Disease in Workhouses: Instructions to Permanent and Temporary Poor Law Inspectors*, p.128.

46. Ibid., Appendix A, No. IX, Circulars, Ophthalmic Diseases in Workhouses: Instructions to Permanent and Temporary Poor Law Inspectors, pp.128–9.

47. *Kanturk Union. Statement of the Number of Persons who have Become Blind, or Who have Lost the Sight of One Eye, in the Workhouses of the Kanturk Union*, BPP, 1852 (265), xlvi, p.4.

48. Scraggs found seventy-four cases of permanent blindness and 180 with loss of sight in one eye on his arrival at the workhouse. Many of the blind had been taken from the house when families left, fearing more of them would be infected with the disease. See *Kanturk Union. Statement of the Number of Persons who have Become Blind, or Who have Lost the Sight of One Eye, in the Workhouses of the Kanturk Union*, BPP 1852 (265), p.9.

49. Ibid., BPP 1852 (265), p.11.

50. Ibid., p.16.

51. Ibid., p.18.

52. C. Ó Gráda and J. Mokyr, 'Famine Disease and Famine Mortality', in C. Ó Gráda (ed.), *Ireland's Great Famine: Interdisciplinary Perspectives* (Dublin: UCD Press, 2006), pp.63–7.

53. In the 1851 Census, in the report on the tables of death during the Famine, it is noted that ophthalmia was recorded instead in the 'table of pestilence' because it was not fatal. *The Census of Ireland for the Year 1851. Part V. Tables of Death, Vol. II. Containing the Report, Tables of Pestilence and Analysis of the Tables and Deaths*, 1856 (2087–II), xxx, p.439.

54. *Report of the Commissioners of Health, Ireland, on the Epidemics of 1846 to 1850*, BPP 1852-3 (1562) xli, pp 25–6. The ophthalmic epidemic is not mentioned in this report. See also C. Kinealy, 'The Poor Law during the Great Famine: An Administration in Crisis', in E.M. Crawford (ed.), *Famine: The Irish Experience, 900–1900* (Edinburgh: John Donald Publishers, 1989), pp.157–75.

55. Kirkpatrick, 'The Epidemic Ophthalmia of the Irish Workhouses', p.8.

56. Wilde, 'On the Epidemic Ophthalmia', p.18.

57. *Twelfth Annual Report of the Commissioners for Administering the Laws for Relief of the Poor in Ireland, with Appendices*, 1859, session 2 (2546), xix, p.149.

58. The asylums were Simpson's Hospital, the Richmond, the Molyneaux, St Mary's and St Joseph's in Dublin, the Macan in Armagh with facilities also in Belfast, Limerick and

Cork. The range of skills included basket, mat and brush-making, knitting, sewing and weaving. Subjects included 'reading on raised letters', arithmetic, history, geography, scripture and music. *The Census of Ireland for the Year 1861. Part III. Vital Statistics. Vol. 1. Report and Tables relating to the Status of Disease.* BPP 1863 (3204–II), lviii, pp.44–5.

59. Ibid., p.150. Fifty children from the Cork Union workhouse were permanently accommodated in the blind asylum in that city. J. Arnott, mayor of Cork, attributed their loss of sight to the poor diet in the workhouse. See J. Arnott, *An Investigation into the Condition of the Children in the Cork Workhouse with an Analysis of the Evidence* (Cork: Guy Brothers, 1859), pp.5–8; *Cork Union Workhouse. Abstract Return. Copy of the Report of the Inspector Appointed to hold an Investigation into the State of the Cork Union Workhouse, in the Months of April and May 1859, and of the Evidence taken before Such Inspector, and of Correspondence Relating Thereto*, BPP 1861 (184), lv, pp.4, 17, 18, 19.

60. E.C. Johnson, *The Irish Pauper Blind: Their Present Condition and Future Prospects*, LSE selected pamphlets (London: Mallett, 1860), p.10.

61. Poor Afflicted Persons Relief (Ireland) Act, 16 August 1878 (41 & 42 Vic., c.60).

62. C.R. Keeler, 'The Ophthalmoscope in the Lifetime of Herman von Helmholtz', *Archives of Ophthalmology*, 120, 2 (2002), pp.194–201.

Chapter 5

1. J. Robins, *Fools and Mad: A History of the Insane in Ireland* (Dublin: Institute of Public Administration, 1986); M. Finanne, *Insanity and the Insane in Post-Famine Ireland* (London: Croom Helm, 1981).

2. J.B. Lyons, *Aspects of History of Medicine in Ireland* (Dublin: Irish Epilepsy Association, 1997), p.21.

3. G. Fealy, *A History of Apprenticeship Nurse Training in Ireland* (London: Routledge, 2005), p.16.

4. H. Andrews, 'Robert J. Graves', in J. McGuire and J. Quinn (eds), *Dictionary of Irish Biography* (Cambridge: Cambridge University Press, 2009), p.163.

5. C. MacDonald, 'The Beginnings of the National Hospital, Queen Square (1859–1860)', *British Medical Journal (BMJ)*, 1, 5189 (Summer 1960), pp.1829–1937.

6. See Lyons, *Aspects of History*, p.24.

7. E.H. Reynolds, 'Robert Bentley Todd (1809–1860)', *Journal of Neurology*, 252, 4 (2005), pp.500–1.

8. R.B. Todd and W. Bowman (eds), *The Physiological Anatomy and Physiology of Man*, vol. 2 (London: John W. Parker, 1856), p.115.

9. See Lyons, *Aspects of History*, p.19.

10. Anon., *The Dublin Examiner, in Anatomy, Physiology, Surgery, Practice of Physic, and the Collateral Branches of Medicine* (Dublin: Fannin & Co., 1846), p.127.

11. This was noted in 1840 and 1861, *Report upon the Tables of Deaths for 1841, House of Commons Papers, Census of Ireland for the Year, 1861, 58*, p.27.

12. R.J. Graves, 'On the Nature and Treatment of Epilepsy', *Dublin Quarterly Journal of Medical Science (DQJMS)*, 14, 27 (1852), pp.258–64.

13. See Anon., *Dublin Examiner*, p.126.

14. Ibid.

15. Graves, 'Nature and Treatment of Epilepsy', pp.258–64.

16. Anon., *Dublin Examiner*, p.129.

17. 14 & 15 Vic., c.68.

18. C. Cox, 'Access and Engagement: The Medical Dispensary Service in Post-Famine Ireland', in C. Cox and M. Luddy (eds), *Cultures of Care in Irish Medical History* (Basingstoke: Palgrave Macmillan, 2010), pp.57–78.

19. Ibid.

20. The full extent of its presence and influence on orthodox medicine in Ireland as well as its religious context is the subject of current research.

21. C. Luther, *Concise View of the System of Homoeopathy and Refutation of the Objections* (Dublin: Fannin & Co., 1845), p.3. See also Rhóda Uí Chonaire, 'The Luther Legacy: Homeopathy in Ireland in the Nineteenth Century', *Journal of the Irish Society of Homeopaths* (2010), pp.17–24.

22. *Quarterly Homoeopathic Journal*, 2, 1 (1850), p.317.

23. Luther, *Concise View*, p.62.

24. W.R. Wilde, *Austria: Its Literary, Scientific, and Medical Institutions* (Dublin: W. Curry Jun. and Co., 1843), p.278; see also Philomena Gorey's chapter in this volume.

25. Anon., *Dublin Examiner*, p.130.

26. Ibid., p.132.

27. F. Churchill, *On the Diseases of Infants and Children* (Philadelphia: Blanchard & Lee, 1856), p.131.

28. J. Neligan, *Medicines, their Use and Mode of Administration*, 3rd edn (New York: Harpur & Brothers, 1859), pp.193–4.

29. W.C. Townsend, 'Case of Scarlatina, followed by Dropsy – Convulsions – Hemiplegia – Recovery in Transactions of the Cork Pathological and Medico-Chirurgical Society', *DQJMS*, 47, 93 (Summer 1869), pp.487–9.

30. Anon., *Dublin Examiner*, p.132.

31. Neligan, *Medicines*, p.47.

32. Anon., *Dublin Examiner*, p.131.

33. Ibid., p.94.

34. H. Newton, 'Children's Physic: Medical Perceptions and Treatment of Sick Children in Early Modern England, c. 1580–1720', *Social History of Medicine*, 23, 3 (2010), pp.456–74, at p.466.

35. Neligan, *Medicines*, p.119.

36. Ibid., p.384.

37. Cox, 'The Medical Marketplace', p.60.

38. Anon., *Dublin Examiner*, p.131.

39. Townsend, 'Case of Scarlatina', pp.487–9.

40. 'Reports of the Pathological Society of Dublin 1852–3', *DQJMS*, 15, 29 (1853), pp.467–82.

41. See case in England of parents who, having read a medical textbook, implored their doctor to use leeches on their 14-month-old daughter who was suffering from suspected cerebral congestion in order to prevent her death, in W.J. Cox, 'On the More Rare Nervous Diseases of Children', *DQJMS*, 35, 69 (Summer 1863), pp.344–52. See also Newton, 'Children's Physic', p.11.

42. R.J. Graves, 'Observations on the Treatment of Various Diseases', *Dublin Journal of Medical Science (DJMS)*, 3, 7 (1833), pp.151–72.

43. 'Reports of the Pathological Society of Dublin 1852–3', pp.473–4.

44. Ibid.

45. See case of 11-year-old boy who underwent the same course of treatment but who fully recovered, in Townsend, 'Case of Scarlatina', p.488.

46. Wilde became editor of the *Dublin Journal of Medical Science* in 1845.

47. B. Crosbie, *Irish Imperial Networks: Migration, Social Communication and Exchange in India* (Cambridge and New York: Cambridge University Press, 2011), p.190.

48. J.B. Lyons, 'William Wilde', in McGuire and Quinn (eds), *Dictionary of Irish Biography*.

49. J. Osborne, 'A Comparative Effect of Some Remedies Used in Epilepsy', *DQJMS*, 22, 44 (1856), pp.337–50.

50. See folk medicine in C. Cox, 'The Medical Marketplace and Medical Tradition in Nineteenth-Century Ireland', in R. Moore and S. McClean (eds), *Folk Healing and Health Care Practices in Britain and Ireland: Stethoscopes, Wands, and Crystals* (Oxford and New York: Berghahn Books, 2010), pp.55–80.

51. W. Pickells, 'Deleterious Practice of Some of the Irish Peasantry Connected with the Belief in Fairies', *Edinburgh Medical and Surgical Journal*, 76, 189 (1851), pp.57–63.

52. Ibid.

53. R.J. Graves, 'On the Nature and Treatment of Epilepsy', *DQJMS*, 14, 27 (1852), pp.258–64.

54. Ibid., p.259.

55. J. Osborne, 'A Comparative Effect of Some Remedies Used in Epilepsy', *DQJMS*, 22, 44 (1856), pp.337–50.

56. At this time, chloroform was also used extensively on infants and children with convulsions and epilepsy in England: see W. Cox, 'More Rare Diseases of Nervous System', pp.344–52. In Ireland, Dr R. Johns contended that chloroform produced epilepsy in women subject to it and caused convulsions in infants: see R. Johns, 'Practical Observations on the Injurious Effects of Chloroform in Labour', *DQJMS* 35, 70 (1863), pp.353–65.

57. See sketches of 'skin eruptions': H. Radcliffe Crocker, 'Eruptions from Bromides and Iodides', *BMJ*, 2, 1718 (Winter 1893), pp.1208–9.

58. J.M. Purser, 'On the Physiological Action of Bromide of Potassium', *DQJMS*, 47, 94 (1869), pp.321–35.

59. Bromide of potassium was mixed with the syrup of bitter orange peel to make it more palatable. While there is no specific reference to the administration of the syrup mixture to children, it seems likely that it was particularly suitable for younger patients. See W.G. Smith, 'Report on Materia Medica and Therapeutics', *DQJMS*, 49, 97 (Winter 1870), pp.207–36.

60. Smith, 'Report on Materia Medica and Therapeutics', pp.207–36.

61. See Dr Armory's findings, ibid., p.220.

62. See cases of adult epilepsy treated with bromides in T. Hayden, 'On the Use of Bromide of Potassium in the Treatment of Epilepsy', *DQJMS*, 57, 26 (1874), pp.151–73.

63. Smith, 'Materia Medica', p.211.

64. 'Digitalis and Bromide of Potassium in Epilepsy', *BMJ*, 1 (1870), p.32.

65. A. Roche, 'The Bromide of Strontium in Epilepsy', *BMJ*, 1, 1794 (Summer 1895), p.1089.

66. S.D. Shorvon, 'The Causes of Epilepsy: Changing Concepts of Etiology of Epilepsy Over the Past 150 years', *Epilepsia*, 52, 6 (2011), pp.1033–44.

67. W. Friedlander, *The History of Modern Epilepsy: The Beginning, 1865-1914* (Westport, CT: Greenwood Press, 2001), p.2.

68. Ibid.

69. Reynolds, 'Robert Bentley Todd', pp.500–1.

70. Friedlander, *History of Modern Epilepsy*, p.113.

71. A. Wynne Foot, 'A Case of Gastric Epilepsy', *Transactions of the Royal Academy of Medicine in Ireland*, 6, 1 (1888), pp.45–55.

72. See neurosurgery in the twentieth century in Lyons, *Aspects of History*, p.29.

73. O. Tempkin, *The Falling Sickness: A History of Epilepsy from the Greeks to the Beginnings of Modern Neurology* (Baltimore and London: The Johns Hopkins University Press, 1945), pp.230–2.

74. T.H. Turner, 'Maudsley, Henry (1835–1918)', *Oxford Dictionary of National Biography* (Oxford: Oxford University Press, 2004).

75. H. Maudsley, 'On Some Causes of Insanity', *British Journal of Psychiatry*, 11 (1867), pp.488–502.

76. C. Lombrosso, *Criminal Man*, trans. M. Gibson and N. Hahn Rafter (Durham, NC: Duke University Press, 2006).

77. R. Noll, *The Encyclopaedia of Schizophrenia and Other Psychotic Disorders* (New York: Infobase Publishing, 1992), p.118.

78. Ibid.

79. Ibid.

80. See Robins, *Fools and Mad*, p.158.

81. Ibid., p.159.

82. Reports by the Resident Physician to the Board of Governors, RDLA, 1861–4, 1863 (NLI, MS 9816).

83. Ibid., 1863.

84. 30 & 31 Vic., c.118.

85. *Report on District, Local and Private Lunatic Asylums in Ireland with appendices 1872*, p.6, H.C. 1873 (852).

86. Admission Registers, 1852–1907 (NAI, RDLA papers, MS 1223/3/21–40).

87. Ibid.

88. *Seventeenth Report on Industrial Schools in Ireland, 1879*, p.9.

89. *The Fortieth Report of the Inspectors of Lunatics in Ireland, 1891*, p.18.

90. See Finnane, *Insanity and the Insane*, p.151.

91. *Census of Ireland for the year 1851, part iii: report of the status of disease 1851*, p.86, H.C. 1854 (1765), liii.

92. R.J. Graves, 'Case of Long-Continued Epilepsy Without any Appreciable Lesion of the Brain or Spinal Marrow', *DJMS*, 17, 51 (1840), pp.373–6.

93. Lyons, *Aspects of History*, p.25.

94. Ibid.

95. *Irish Times*, 24 June 1870.

96. Ibid.

97. See Robins, *Fools and Mad*, p.137.

98. J. Lalor, 'On the Use of Education and Training in the Treatment of the Insane in Public Lunatic Asylums', *Journal of Statistical and Social Inquiry of Ireland*, 7, 54 (1878), pp.361–73, at pp.361–2.

99. Annual Report, RDLA, 1878 (NLI), p.7.

100. Female Case Book, 1887–8 (NAI, RDLA, MS 1223), p.226.

101. See Finnane, *Insanity and the Insane*, p.203.

102. Ibid., pp.191–2.

103. Ibid., p.206.

104. C. Norman, 'The Domestic Treatment of the Insane', *Transactions of the Royal Academy of Medicine in Ireland*, 13, 1 (1895), pp.412–26.

105. *The Fortieth Report of the Inspectors of Lunatics in Ireland, 1891*, p.197.

106. See Fealy, *Apprenticeship Nurse Training*, p.14.

107. Á. Hyland and K. Milne (eds), *Irish Educational Documents*, vol. 2 (Dublin: CICE, 1992), p.460.

108. See Robins, *Fools and Mad*, p.167.

109. Annual Report, RDLA, 1881 (NLI).

110. See Robins, *Fools and Mad*, p.139.

111. Minutes of Meetings (NAI, RDLA papers, MS 1223/1/14), p.168.

112. Ibid.

113. See Robins, *Fools and Mad*, p.167.

114. Male Case Book, 1885–7 (NAI, RDLA papers, MS 1223), pp.80–3.

115. Ibid.

116. Ibid.

117. Ibid.

118. Ibid.

119. Ibid.

120. Ibid.

121. Female Case Book, 1903-4 (NAI, RDLA papers, MS 1223), pp.422–3.

122. Ibid.

123. Ibid.

124. Ibid.

125. Ibid.

126. Ibid.

127. Ibid.

128. Ibid.

129. J. Reynolds, *Grangegorman: Psychiatric Care in Dublin since 1815* (Dublin: Institute of Public Administration, 1992), p.112.

130. See Robins, *Fools and Mad*, p.112.

131. Annual Reports, RDLA, 1870–90 (NLI).

132. Female Case Book, 1902–3 (NAI, RDLA papers, MS 1223), p.445.

133. Ibid., p.104.

134. Ibid., p.85.

135. Ibid., p.104.

136. The Medico-Psychological Association of Great Britain and Ireland, *BMJ*, 2, 2642 (Summer 1911), pp.396–7.

137. L. Symes, 'On the Mortality of Children in Ireland, 1886–1896', *Transactions of the Royal Academy of Medicine in Ireland*, 16, 1 (1898), pp.381–95.

138. Ibid., pp.389–90.

139. See Symes, 'Mortality of Children', pp.381–95.

140. Ibid., p.393.

141. See Finnane, *Insanity and the Insane*, p.187.

Chapter 6

1. *Twenty-Ninth Report of the Inspectors-General on the General State of the Prisons in Ireland*, Commons, Reports of Commissioners, Command Papers, 1851 [1364], xxviii.357, p.xix.

2. Ibid., p.xx.

3. M. May, 'Innocence and Experience: The Evolution of the Concept of Juvenile Delinquency in the Mid-Nineteenth Century', *Victorian Studies*, 17, 1 (September 1973), pp.7–29.

4. J. Calder, *The Victorian Home* (London: Book Club Associates, 1977), pp.155. See also J. Bourke, *Husbandry to Housewifery: Women, Economic Change and Housework in Ireland, 1890–1914* (Oxford and New York: Oxford University Press, 1993).

5. J. Duckworth, *Fagin's Children: Criminal Children in Victorian England* (London: Hambledon & London, 2002), p.19.

6. G. Himmelfarb, *The Idea of Poverty: England in the Early Industrial Age* (London and Boston: Faber & Faber, 1984), pp.326–7, 367, 395; D. Taylor, 'Beyond the Bounds of Respectable Society: The "Dangerous Classes" in Victorian and Edwardian England', in J. Rowbotham and K. Stevenson (eds), *Criminal Conversations: Victorian Crimes, Social Panic and Moral Outrage* (Columbus, OH: Ohio State University Press, 2005), pp.3–22.

7. M. Weiner, *Reconstructing the Criminal: Culture, Law and Policy in England, 1830–1914* (Cambridge: Cambridge University Press, 1990), pp.33–5.

8. Ibid., pp.26–36; D. Pick, *Faces of Degeneration: A European Disorder, c. 1848–1918* (Cambridge: Cambridge University Press, 1989), pp.176–203.

9. J. Barnes, *Irish Industrial Schools, 1868–1908: Expansion and Development* (Dublin: Irish Academic Press, 1989), p.17.

10. T. Feeney, 'Church, State and Family: The Advent of Child Guidance Clinics in Independent Ireland', *Social History of Medicine*, 25, 4 (October 2012), pp.848-62.

11. M. Luddy, *Women and Philanthropy in Nineteenth-Century Ireland* (Cambridge: Cambridge University Press, 1995), pp.68–96.

12. *Commission to Inquire into Child Abuse, Volumes 1–5* (Dublin: Stationery Office, 2009).

13. M. Rafferty and E. O'Sullivan, *Suffer the Little Children: The Inside Story of Ireland's Industrial Schools* (Dublin: New Island, 1999).

14. C. Reidy, *Ireland's 'Moral Hospital': The Irish Borstal System, 1906–56* (Dublin: Irish Academic Press, 2009).

15. M. Daly, *Dublin, the Deposed Capital: A Social and Economic History, 1860–1914* (Cork: Cork University Press, 1985), pp.77–81; C. Breathnach, *The Congested Districts Board, 1891–1923: Poverty and Development in the West of Ireland* (Dublin: Four Courts Press, 2005).

16. 'Irish Convict Prisons', *Dublin University Magazine*, 51, 1 (February 1858), pp.166–72.

17. J. Taylor, *Amalgamation of Unions, and Pauper and National Education in Ireland* (Dublin: John Falconer, 1857), p.115.

18. J. Abbott, 'The Press and the Public Visibility of Nineteenth-Century Criminal Children', in Rowbotham and Stevenson (eds), *Criminal Conversations*, pp.23–39.

19. *Irish Times*, 9 July 1861. See also M. O'Brien, 'Journalism in Ireland: The Evolution of a Discipline', in K. Rafter (ed.), *Irish Journalism before Independence: More a Disease than a Profession* (Manchester: Manchester University Press, 2010), pp.22–35.

20. S. Magarey, 'The Invention of Juvenile Delinquency in Early Nineteenth-Century England', *Labour History*, 34 (May 1978), pp.11–27; P. King, *Crime and Law in England, 1750–1840: Remaking Justice from the Margins* (Cambridge: Cambridge University Press, 2006), p.113.

21. *Thirty-First Report of the Inspectors-General on the General State of the Prisons in Ireland*, Command Papers, Reports of Commissioners, 1852–3 [1657], vol. liii.1, pp.21–2.

22. *Thirty-Fifth Report of the Inspectors-General on the General State of the Prisons in Ireland*, Command Papers, Reports of Commissioners, 1857 [2236], vol. xxii.173, p.xxxviii.

23. Carpenter was cited copiously in the annual reports of the inspectors of reformatory schools in Ireland. See for instance *Second Report of the Inspector Appointed to Visit the Reformatory Schools of Ireland*, Command Papers, Reports of Commissioners, 1863 [3194], vol. xxiv.623, pp.14–18.

24. M. Carpenter, *Juvenile Delinquents: Their Condition and Treatment* (London: W. & F.G. Cash, 1853), p.15.

25. Ibid., pp.15–16.

26. Ibid., pp.293–4.

27. Ibid., p.163.

28. M. Ignatieff, *A Just Measure of Pain: The Penitentiary in the Industrial Revolution 1750–1850* (London: Macmillan Press, 1978).

29. G.S. Frost, *Victorian Childhoods* (Westport, CT: Praeger, 2009), pp.133–4.

30. May, 'Innocence and Experience'.

31. P.J. Murray, *Reformatories in Ireland, and for Dublin in Particular* (Dublin: W.B. Kelly, 1858), pp.1, xlvi.

32. J. Haughton, 'The Social and Moral Elevation of our People', *Journal of the Dublin Statistical Society*, 3, 3 (July 1857), pp.63–72.

33. M. O'Shaughnessy, 'The Educational and other Aspects of the Statistics of Crime in Dublin', *Journal of the Statistical and Social Inquiry Society of Ireland*, 3, 2 (May 1861), pp.61–70.

34. T.M. Madden, *On Insanity and the Criminal Responsibility of the Insane* (Dublin: John Falconer, 1866), p.7.

35. Ibid., pp.8–9.

36. Reformatory Schools (Ireland) Act, 1858 (21 & 22 Vic., c.103; Industrial Schools Act (Ireland), 1868 (31 & 32 Vic., c.25).

37. *Commission to Inquire into Child Abuse*, vol. 1 (Dublin: Stationery Office, 2009), p.36.

38. Ibid., p.38.

39. P. Carroll-Burke, *Colonial Discipline: The Making of the Irish Convict System* (Dublin: Four Courts Press, 2000), pp.113–14.

40. W.N. Hancock, 'The Aberdeen Industrial Schools Contrasted with Irish Workhouses: Family Ties Being Cherished in the Schools and Violated in the Workhouses', *Journal of the Statistical and Social Inquiry Society of Ireland*, 3, 28 (January 1861), pp.6–18.

41. E. Leaney, 'John Francis O'Neill Lentaigne', in *Dictionary of Irish Biography*. Accessed 27 April 2012, 15.24 p.m, <http://dib.cambridge.org/viewReadPage.do?articleId=a4795&searchClicked=clicked&searchBy=1&browsesearch=yes>.

42. Barnes, *Irish Industrial Schools*, pp.51–4.

43. *Second Report of the Inspector*, p.41.

44. Ibid., p.43.

45. *Tenth Report of the Inspector Appointed to Visit the Reformatory and Industrial Schools of Ireland*, BPP 1872 [671] xxx, p.51.

46. *Fourteenth Report of the Inspector Appointed to Visit the Reformatory and Industrial Schools of Ireland*, BPP 1876 [494], xxxiv, p.22.

47. M. Finnane, *Insanity and the Insane in Nineteenth-Century Ireland* (London: Croom Helm, 1981), pp.190–201.

48. *Ninth Report of the Inspector Appointed to Visit the Reformatory and Industrial Schools of Ireland*, BPP 1871 [461] xxviii, p.25.

49. *Second Report of the Inspector*, p.16.

50. R. Carmichael, *An Essay on the Nature of Scrofula* (London: John Callow, 1810), p.39.

51. B. Phillips, *Scrofula: Its Nature, Its Causes, Its Prevalence and the Principles of Treatment* (Philadelphia: Lea & Blanchard, 1846), pp.178–86.

52. *Tenth Report of the Inspector*, p.71.

53. *Eleventh Report of the Inspector Appointed to Visit the Reformatory and Industrial Schools of Ireland*, BPP 1873 [858] xxxi, p.30.

54. M. Foucault, *Discipline and Punish* (New York: Pantheon Books, 1977).

55. *Fourteenth Report of the Inspector*, p.22; F. von Niemeyer, trans. G.H. Humphreys and C. E. Hackley, *A Text-Book of Practical Medicine, with Particular Reference to Physiology and Pathological Anatomy* (New York: D. Appleton & Co., 1869), p.745.

56. *Tenth Report of the Inspector*, p.45.

57. *Ninth Report of the Inspector*, p.21.

58. *Tenth Report of the Inspector*, p.45.

59. *Eleventh Report of the Inspector*, p.20.

60. For comparison with other institutional diets, see I. Miller, *Reforming Food in Post-Famine Ireland: Medicine, Science and Improvement, 1845-1922* (Manchester: Manchester University Press, forthcoming), Chapter 3.

61. For more on the relationship between contemporary ideas on diet and national well-being, see I. Miller, *A Modern History of the Stomach: Gastric Illness, Medicine, and British Society, 1800-1950* (London: Pickering and Chatto, 2011), pp.11-38.

62. See ibid.

63. See, for instance, criticism raised in W.N. Hancock, 'On the Mortality of Children in Workhouses in Ireland', *Journal of the Statistical and Social Inquiry Society of Ireland*, 3, 3 (June 1862), pp.193–7 and J. Arnott, *The Investigation into the Condition of the Children in the Cork Workhouse* (Cork: Guy Brothers, 1859).

64. *Ninth Report of the Inspector*, p.21.

65. *Annual Report of the Commissioners for Administering the Laws for the Relief of the Poor in Ireland*, BPP 1871 [361] xxviii, p.19.

66. R.B. Carter, *A Practical Treatise on Diseases of the Eye* (London: Macmillan and Co., 1875), p.216; *Fourteenth Report of the Inspector*, p.108.

67. *Eighteenth Report of the Inspector Appointed to Visit the Reformatory and Industrial Schools of Ireland*, BPP 1880 [2692] xxxvii, p.70.

68. M. Worboys, *Spreading Germs: Diseases, Theories and Medical Practice in Britain, 1865–1900* (Cambridge: Cambridge University Press, 2000), p.288.

69. Ibid., p.62.

70. *Nineteenth Report of the Inspector Appointed to Visit the Reformatory and Industrial Schools of Ireland*, BPP 1881 [3070] liii, p.18.

71. Ibid.

72. *The Times*, 22 April 1882; *Twentieth Report of the Inspector Appointed to Visit the Reformatory and Industrial Schools of Ireland*, BPP 1882 [3372] xxxv, p.21.

73. See H. Hendrick, 'Child Labour, Medical Capital and the School Medical Service, c. 1890–1918', in R. Cooter (ed.), *In the Name of the Child: Health and Welfare, 1880–1940* (London and New York: Routledge, 1992), pp.45–71.

74. *Twenty-Seventh Report of the Inspector Appointed to Visit the Reformatory and Industrial Schools of Ireland*, BPP 1889 [5858] xlii, p.15.

75. *Twenty-Eighth Report of the Inspector Appointed to Visit the Reformatory and Industrial Schools of Ireland*, BPP 1890 [6168] xxxvii, part 1, p.13.

Chapter 7

1. D. Price, 'Tuberculosis in Adolescents', *Irish Journal of Medical Science (IJMS)*, 6, 159 (1939), p.129.

2. G. Jones, '"Captain of all These Men of Death": The History of Tuberculosis in Nineteenth- and Twentieth-Century Ireland' (Amsterdam: Rodopi, 2001), p.2. In this chapter, Ireland, prior to 1922, refers to the thirty-two counties while Ireland, post 1922, refers to the twenty-six counties.

3. Ibid., p.2; J. Deeny, 'The Present State of Human Tuberculosis in Ireland', *Journal of the Statistical and Social Inquiry Society of Ireland (JSSISI)*, 20, 5 (1961/2), p.130.

4. J.E. Counihan and T.W.T. Dillon, 'Irish Tuberculosis Death Rates: A Statistical Study of their Reliability, with some Socio-Economic Conditions', *JSSISI*, 17, 5 (1943/4), p.169.

5. Counihan and Dillon, 'Irish Tuberculosis Death Rates', p.169; R.J. Rowlette, 'Tuberculosis in Éire', *IJMS*, 6, 199 (1942), pp.221–43; also cited in Jones, *'Captain of all These Men of Death'*, p.136.

6. T. McKeown, *The Modern Rise of Population* (London: Edward Arnold, 1976), p.153.

7. See for instance: S. Szreter, 'Economic Growth, Disruption, Deprivation, Disease and Death: On the Importance of the Politics of Public Health for Development', *Population and Development Review*, 23, 4 (1997), pp 693–728; F.B. Smith, *The Retreat of Tuberculosis, 1850–1950* (London, New York and Sydney: Croom Helm, 1988); L. Bryder, *Below the Magic Mountain: A Social History of Tuberculosis in Twentieth-Century Britain* (Oxford: Oxford University Press, 1988); N. McFarlane, 'Hospitals, Housing and Tuberculosis in Glasgow, 1911–51', *Social History of Medicine (SHM)*, 2, 1 (1989), pp.59–85; G.D. Feldberg, *Disease and Class: Tuberculosis and the Shaping of Modern North American Society* (New Brunswick, NJ: Rutgers University Press, 1995); M. Niemi, *Public Health and Municipal Policy Making: Britain and Sweden, 1900–1940* (Aldershot and Burlington, VT: Ashgate, 2007); M. Gandy, 'Life without Germs', in M.

Gandy and A. Zumla (eds), *The Return of the White Plague: Global Poverty and the 'New' Tuberculosis* (London and New York: Verso, 2003), pp.15–38; P. Weindling, 'From Germ Theory to Social Medicine', in D. Brunton (ed.), *Medicine Transformed: Health, Disease and Society in Europe, 1800–1930* (Manchester: Manchester University Press, 2004), pp.239–65.

8. Jones, *'Captain of all These Men of Death'*.

9. See also Susan Kelly's chapter in this volume.

10. D. Price, *Tuberculosis in Childhood* (Bristol: Wright & Sons, 1942), pp.1–5; *Annual Reports of the Registrar General, 1926–1955* (National Library of Ireland (NLI), T3/6–35). The reports of the registrar general consistently show that the percentage of tubercular deaths in children under 15 years of age due to non-pulmonary tuberculosis outnumbered those caused by pulmonary tuberculosis. Miliary tuberculosis was most commonly associated with children but could, in rare cases, affect adults.

11. *Annual Reports of the Registrar General, 1922–1955; Department of Health Annual Reports on Vital Statistics, 1956–67* (NLI, T1/6–46, U3/66–7). Death rates in children largely fell in line with overall death rates; however, there were divergences, as shown in the table below, which is derived from the annual reports. Death rates from tuberculosis at different ages per 1,000 population (Ireland):

Period	Under 15	15–19	20–24	25–34	35–44	45–54	55 & over	All ages
1925–27	0.72	1.82	2.63	2.58	2.07	1.56	0.81	1.50
1935–37	0.53	1.36	2.25	2.18	1.63	1.32	0.71	1.22
1945–47	0.52	1.40	2.17	1.99	1.58	1.38	0.87	1.22
1948–50	0.34	0.78	1.46	1.54	1.29	1.20	0.75	0.92
1955–57	0.07	0.06	0.16	0.29	0.34	0.41	0.51	0.26
1960–62	0.02	0.01	0.04	0.10	0.20	0.25	0.40	0.16
1964–66	0.01	0.01	0.01	0.06	0.13	0.19	0.39	0.12
1965–67	0.01	0.01	0.01	0.03	0.10	0.16	0.35	0.11

12. J. Prunty, *Dublin Slums, 1800–1925: A Study in Urban Geography* (Dublin: Irish Academic Press, 1998), p.234; see also Laura Kelly's chapter in this volume.

13. M. Dunlevy, 'Medical and Social Problems of Childhood Tuberculosis in Dublin', *Journal of the Medical Association of Éire (JMAÉ)*, 23, 134 (1948), p.19; M. Dunlevy, 'Lowered Tuberculosis Death Rates in Dublin Children', *JMAÉ*, 24, 142 (1949), p.56.

14. R. Collis, *The State of Medicine in Ireland* (Dublin: Parkside Press, 1943), p.49; see also Susan Kelly's chapter in this volume. Collis pointed out that many infants dying of

tuberculosis were diagnosed as 'marasmus, enteritis, etc.', while many death certificates were unreliable due to some insurance companies refusing to pay burial insurance if the death was due to tuberculosis, on the grounds that tuberculosis was a hereditary disease.

15. V.M. Synge, 'Introduction', in L. Price, *Dorothy Price: An Account of Twenty Years' Fight against Tuberculosis in Ireland* (Oxford: Oxford University Press, 1957), p.v. For private circulation only.

16. J.A. Lunn, 'Practical Issues of Tuberculin Testing', *Practitioner*, 227, 1376 (1983), pp.xiv–vi.

17. M. Crowe, 'Local Authority Tuberculosis Schemes: Suggestions for their Better Development', *IJMS*, 6, 33 (1945), p.154; J. Duffy, 'Review of Pulmonary Tuberculosis in Practice', *Journal of the Irish Free State Medical Union (JIFSMU)*, 1, 6 (1937), p.72; White Paper, *Tuberculosis*, Official publication P.7368 (Dublin: Stationery Office, 1946), p.16; J.A. Deeny, 'Aspects of the Problem in Éire', *IJMS*, 6, 252 (1946), p.774; J. Deeny, *To Cure and to Care: Memoirs of a Chief Medical Officer* (Dun Laoghaire: Glendale Publishing), pp.99–100. Crowe asserted that sputum testing was also neglected. John Duffy, an assistant County Medical Officer of Health (CMOH) in the tuberculosis service, noted that 'of the vitally important early development of the disease' he learned 'little or nothing' from his teachers or textbooks. The 1946 White Paper recorded a lack of hospital laboratories and X-ray equipment.

18. See Susan Kelly's chapter in this volume.

19. Jones, *'Captain of all These Men of Death'*, pp.145, 157; M. Ó hÓgartaigh, 'Dr Dorothy Price and the Elimination of Childhood Tuberculosis', in J. Augusteijn (ed.), *Ireland in the 1930s: New Perspectives* (Dublin: Four Courts Press, 1999), pp.76–7; M. Ó hÓgartaigh, 'Dorothy Stopford-Price and the Elimination of Childhood Tuberculosis', in M. Ó hÓgartaigh (ed.), *Quiet Revolutionaries: Irish Women in Education, Medicine and Sport, 1861–1964* (Dublin: The History Press, 2011), pp.106–20; R. Barrington, *Health, Medicine and Politics in Ireland, 1900–1970* (Dublin: Institute of Public Administration, 1987), p.130; L. Bryder, F. Condrau and M. Worboys, 'Tuberculosis and its Histories: Then and Now', in F. Condrau and M. Worboys (eds), *Tuberculosis Then and Now: Perspectives on the History of an Infectious Disease* (Montreal, Kingston, London and Ithaca: McGill-Queen's University Press, 2010), pp.3–23. Bryder, Condrau and Worboys' comprehensive overview of the historiography demonstrates the lack of emphasis, to date, placed on tuberculin testing as an intervention in disease control both at individual and population level. In the Irish context, Ó hÓgartaigh discusses Dorothy Price's use of tuberculin while Jones discusses tuberculin testing in the context of emigration.

20. Price, *Tuberculosis in Childhood*, p.v. Without tuberculin testing and radiological examination, a child could be 'condemned to months of inactivity on account of

conditions that are non-tuberculous' or they might suffer 'another distressing picture' where primary tuberculosis is not recognised and the child is 'denied the rest necessary'.

21. Hardy, 'Reframing Disease', p.535.

22. T. Brock, *Robert Koch: A Life in Medicine and Bacteriology* (Washington: ASM Press, 1999), pp.295–313.

23. W.S. Richmond, 'Professor Koch's Remedy for Tuberculosis', *Lancet*, 136, 3512 (1890), pp.1354–5; also cited in Smith, *The Retreat of Tuberculosis*, p.57; H.J. Parish, *A History of Immunisation* (Edinburgh and London: E. and F. Livingstone, 1965), p.111; R. Koch, 'On the New Tuberculin Preparation', trans. H.E. Littledale, *Dublin Journal of Medical Science (DJMS)*, 105, 317 (1898), pp.433–40. Smith quoted the 'grumbler' Dr W.S. Richmond declaring that 'British doctors had no right to inject into patients a secret foreign fluid with nasty side-effects'.

24. S.R. Rosenthal, 'Tuberculin Sensitivity and BCG Vaccination', in S.R. Rosenthal (ed.), *BCG Vaccine: Tuberculosis, Cancer* (Littleton, MA: PSG Publishing Company, 1980), pp.183–4; Brock, *Koch*, p.211. Brock cites Koch's statement that his new remedy was 'nothing more or less than a glycerine extract of a pure culture of tubercle bacilli'. Glycerine was a component of the culture medium used to grow the bacilli.

25. R. Dubos and J. Dubos, *The White Plague: Tuberculosis, Man and Society* (New Brunswick, NJ: Rutgers University Press, 1952), p.106.

26. See for instance: T.M. Healy, *From Sanitorium to Hospital: A Social and Medical Account of Peamount, 1912-1997* (Dublin: A. & A. Farmar, 2002), pp.30–1; G.J. Blackmore, 'Correspondence', *British Medical Journal (BMJ)*, 1, 3760 (1933), pp.164–5; F.E. Gunter, 'Correspondence', *BMJ*, 1, 3760 (1933), pp.164–5.

27. R. Wagner, *Clemens von Pirquet: His Life and Work* (Baltimore: Johns Hopkins University Press, 1968). Von Pirquet (1874–1929) was a clinical assistant at the Kinderklinik in Vienna (1903–9). He was Professor of Paediatrics at the University of Vienna (1911–29).

28. Wagner, *Clemens von Pirquet*, pp.26–7. The Mantoux text was developed in 1908 by the French physician Charles Mantoux.

29. Wagner, *Clemens von Pirquet*, pp.66–9.

30. Elinor Dorothy Stopford (1890–1954) married District Justice Liam Price in 1925. Using the name Dorothy Price, she published widely on childhood tuberculosis in the Irish and British medical literature from 1930 to 1954. She worked in St Ultan's Infant Hospital, Dublin, becoming the first chairwoman of the Irish National BCG Committee; Price, *Dorothy Price*, pp.3–4. The first ten pages of this book were written by Dorothy Price prior to her death in 1954.

31. Professor Edmond Joseph McWeeney (1864–1925), known as EJ, was a Dublin-based pathologist and bacteriologist who had studied in Vienna and Berlin under

Rokitansky and Koch; see also Philomena Gorey's chapter in this volume. The ophthalmologist William Wilde studied in the Allgemeines Krankenhaus in Vienna in the 1840s.

32. Smith, *The Retreat of Tuberculosis*, pp.58–9.

33. J. Gibbens, 'Correspondence', *BMJ*, 1, 3655 (1931), p.156.

34. Ibid.; John Mowbray, 'Growth and Development of Paediatrics in Ireland', *Journal of the Irish Medical Association (JIMA)*, LX, 365 (1967), p.404. The *British Journal of Diseases of Children* was launched in 1904, the first chair of paediatrics was instituted in 1906 at King's College, London, while the British Paediatric Association was set up in 1928.

35. L. Findlay, 'Pulmonary Tuberculosis in Childhood', *Postgraduate Medical Journal*, 9, 96 (1933), p.380.

36. E.J. McWeeney, 'Discussion following Albert Calmette's paper in Belfast', *BMJ*, 2, 2539 (1909), p.530; G.B. M'Hutchison, 'Calmette's Opthalmo-Reaction to Tuberculin', *DJMS*, 126, 439 (1908), pp.16–35. Other early-published studies in Ireland attempted to assess the usefulness of tuberculin as a vaccine or a therapeutic agent.

37. L. Bryder, '"Wonderlands of Buttercup, Clover and Daisies": Tuberculosis and the Open-Air Movement in Britain, 1907–39', in Roger Cooter (ed.), *In the Name of the Child: Health and Welfare, 1880–1940* (London and New York: Routledge, 1992), pp.104–6. Similar tuberculin testing trials, including conjunctival testing, carried out in America in 1908 and 1909, were the subject of enormous controversy, arousing the ire of a number of anti-vivisection societies.

38. The Easter Rising of 1916 was followed by the War of Independence (1919–21) and the Civil War (1922–3).

39. *Department of Local Government and Public Health, First Report 1922–1925* (NLI, K24/1), pp 26–7.

40. Synge, 'Introduction', in Price, *Dorothy Price*, p.v; Price, *Dorothy Price*, p.6; also cited in Ó hÓgartaigh, 'Dr Dorothy', pp.75–6.

41. Wagner, *Clemens von Pirquet*, pp.205–6. Von Pirquet had worked in the clinic but was dead in 1931.

42. Price, *Dorothy Price*, p.1; Dorothy Price enrolled in four courses in the Kinderklinik: surgery in infants, diabetes in children, feeding in infants, and skin. Tuberculosis was not foremost among her interests at this time.

43. Price, *Dorothy Price*, pp.2–3.

44. See Laura Kelly's chapter in this volume for further information on St Ultan's Hospital.

45. Price, *Dorothy Price*, p.5; also cited in Ó hÓgartaigh, 'Dr Dorothy', p.76.

46. Dorothy Price to Liam Price, letter, 3 September 1934 (Trinity College Dublin (TCD), Price Papers, MS 7534/61).

47. D. Price, 'Tuberculosis in infants', *BMJ*, 1, 4022 (1938), pp.275–7.

48. G.B. Fleming, 'Incidence and Treatment of Tuberculosis in Children', *Lancet*, 242, 6271 (1943), p.580.

49. R. Collis (1900–75) was a paediatrician with extensive experience outside Ireland including a stint at the Hospital for Sick Children, Great Ormond Street, London, and Johns Hopkins in Baltimore, USA. His Irish appointments included physician to the National Children's Hospital, Dublin, and Director of Paediatrics in the Rotunda Hospital, Dublin.

50. Price, *Dorothy Price*, pp.3, 9; also cited in Ó hÓgartaigh, 'Dr Dorothy', p.77. Peamount had been founded in 1912 by Lady Aberdeen and the Women's National Health Association.

51. Wallgren experimented with tuberculin testing and BCG vaccination in order to prevent tuberculosis in children. He was chief physician (1921–42) in the Gothenburg Children's Hospital, which was Sweden's largest children's hospital. From 1942 to 1956, he held the Chair of Paediatrics at the Karolinska Institute, Stockholm and was also chief physician of the Norrtull's Children's Hospital which merged with the Karolinska in 1951.

52. Collis later became the English-language editor of Wallgren and Guidi Fanconi's book *Lehrbuch der Pediatrie*, republished in English as *Fanconi and Wallgren's Textbook of Paediatrics* (London: William Heinemann, 1952).

53. Niemi, *Public Health and Municipal Policy Making*, p.187. Niemi contrasts public health and policy-making in Gothenburg in Sweden and Birmingham in Great Britain.

54. D. Price, 'Tuberculosis in Infants', pp.275–7.

55. G.P.G. Beckett to Price, letter, 14 February 1938 (TCD, Price Papers, MS 7534/245).

56. *Department of Local Government and Public Health Report, 1936–1937* (NLI, K24/13), p.174.

57. 'Doctor's Plan to Lower T.B. Rate', *Irish Press*, 13 April 1939.

58. A. Wallgren, 'Combating Tuberculosis in a Swedish City', *IJMS*, 6, 163 (1939), p.292.

59. Price to Wallgren, draft letter, 6 April 1940 (TCD, Price Papers, MS 7535/124).

60. Dr Bastabal, County Donegal, to Price, letter, 23 September 1940 (TCD, Price Papers, MS 7535/136); C. Cox, 'Access and Engagement: The Medical Dispensary Service in Post-Famine Ireland', in C. Cox and M. Luddy (eds), *Cultures of Care in Irish Medical History, 1750–1970* (Basingstoke: Palgrave Macmillan, 2010), pp.57–78.

61. Dorothy Price to the Secretary, Department of Local Government and Public Health, copy of letter, 24 September 1943 (TCD, Price Papers, MS 7536/404).

62. Price, *Tuberculosis in Childhood*, 1st edn, p.138.

63. A. Hardy, *The Epidemic Streets: Infectious Disease and the Rise of Preventive Medicine, 1856–1900* (Oxford: Clarendon Press, 1993), pp.226–7.

64. M. Worboys, *Spreading Germs: Diseases, Theories and Medical Practice in Britain* (Cambridge and New York: Cambridge University Press, 2006), pp.193–4.

65. R. Collis, correspondence, *JMAÉ*, 16, 91 (1945), p.11.

66. M. Dunlevy, 'Medical and Social Problems of Childhood Tuberculosis in Dublin', p.19.

67. W.F. Gaisford, 'Primary Tuberculosis in Childhood', *BMJ*, 1, 4437(1946), p.84.

68. D. Price, 'A Report of Tuberculin Skin Tests in Children', *IJMS*, 6, 103 (1934), pp.302–4.

69. D. Price and T.G. Hardman, 'Tuberculin Skin Reactions', *IJMS*, 6, 105 (1934), pp.540–1.

70. Price, 'Tuberculosis in Adolescents', pp.124–9.

71. D. Price, 'Report of a Tuberculin Survey amongst Children in Dublin Hospitals made by the Irish Paediatric Association', *IJMS*, 6, 187 (1941), pp.241–55.

72. P. Alston, 'Tuberculin Survey in an Industrial School, County Dublin, January–March 1945', *IJMS*, 6, 244 (1946), pp.130–3.

73. P.F. Fitzpatrick, 'A Tuberculosis Contact Survey', *IJMS*, 6, 241 (1946), pp.33–5.

74. M. Grimes, N. Hayes, M. Murphy and L. Bean T. De Barra, 'Statistical Analysis and Results of a Tuberculin Survey carried out in Cork City and County, 1944–46', *IJMS*, 6, 256 (1946), pp.154–70.

75. P.F. Fitzpatrick, 'Some Considerations on Case-Finding', *IJMS*, 6, 281 (1949), p.221.

76. Gaisford, 'Primary Tuberculosis in Childhood', p.84.

77. F.R.G. Heaf, 'Present Trends in Tuberculosis', *IJMS*, 6, 252 (1946), pp.772–3.

78. D. Price, 'Hospital Treatment for Tuberculous Children', *JIFSMU*, 3, 14 (1938), p.23.

79. Jones, *'Captain of all These Men of Death'*, p.188.

80. J.B. Lyons, 'Tuberculin Sensitivity: A Review', *JIMA*, 29, 171 (1951), p.65. Thirteen studies are cited.

81. *Annual Reports of the Registrar General, 1926–1958* (NLI, T3/6–38).

82. D. Price, 'A Tuberculin Survey in Ireland', *IJMS*, 6, 314 (1952), p.85.

83. M. Dunlevy, 'Childhood Tuberculosis in the Mid-Century Decade', *JIMA*, 44, 261 (1959), pp.76–81.

84. M. Dunlevy, 'Vagaries of BCG-Induced Tuberculin Allergy', *Postgraduate Medical Journal*, 40, 460 (1964), p.82.

85. E. Lee and R.S. Holzman, 'Evolution and Current Use of the Tuberculin Test', *Clinical Infectious Diseases*, 34, 3 (2002), pp.365–70.

86. Health Protection Surveillance Centre, *Tuberculosis Guidelines 2010* (Dublin: Health Protection Surveillance Centre, 2010), p.88.

87. 'TB Screening begins at Cork School', *Irish Times*, 23 August 2010; 'Cork Children to be Retested for TB', *Irish Times*, 16 September 2010.

Chapter 8

1. Acknowledgements: I am very grateful to Kathy Purcell, Director of the Airfield Trust, who kindly allowed me access to the Overend Archive at the Airfield Trust, Dublin. Thanks also to Kathleen McEntee of the Children's Sunshine Home. I am also thankful to Dr Sarah-Anne Buckley and the anonymous referees and the editors who all provided valuable feedback which greatly improved the chapter.

2. L.A. Clarkson and E. Margaret Crawford, *Feast and Famine: Food and Nutrition in Ireland, 1500–1920* (Oxford: Oxford University Press, 2001), p.178. 'Country without Cripples', *Irish Times*, 2 June 1930. Clarkson and Crawford have commented that in the period 1500–1920 'rickets does not seem to have been a serious problem in Ireland'. However, an article published in 1930 in the *Irish Times* reported on the fact that 'the cripple problem' in the Irish Free State had 'come to be regarded as a national problem'.

3. 'Lack of Calcium Doubled Rickets Incidence', *Irish Independent*, 7 August 1948; W.E. Jessop, 'Results of Rickets Surveys in Dublin' in 'The Irish National Nutritional Survey', *British Journal of Nutrition*, 4, 2-3 (1950), pp.289–92.

4. I. Robertson, J.A. Ford, W.B. McIntosh and M.G. Dunnigan, 'The Role of Cereals in the Aetiology of Nutritional Rickets: The Lesson of the Irish National Nutritional Survey, 1943–8', *British Journal of Nutrition*, 45, 1 (1981), pp.17–22.

5. Jessop, 'Results of Rickets Surveys in Dublin', p.291.

6. Ibid., pp.289–90.

7. Ibid., p.291.

8. The research for the chapter is largely based on material in the Overend Archive at the Airfield Trust, Dublin, which contains letters, annual reports and photographs relating to the early history of the Children's Sunshine Home.

9. For more on the involvement of Irish women doctors in child health and welfare, see M. Ó hÓgartaigh, *Kathleen Lynn: Irishwoman, Patriot, Doctor* (Dublin: Irish Academic Press, 2006); A. Mac Lellan, '"That Preventable and Curable Disease": Dr Dorothy Price and the Eradication of Tuberculosis in Ireland, 1930–1960' (unpublished PhD thesis, University College Dublin, 2011); and L. Kelly, *Irish Women in Medicine, c. 1880s–1920s: Origins, Education and Careers* (Manchester: Manchester University Press, 2012).

10. J. Prunty, *Dublin Slums, 1800–1925: A Study in Urban Geography* (Dublin: Irish Academic Press, 1998), p.272.

11. Prunty has argued that the intensity of the public 'battle for bodies and souls' between Protestant and Catholic charitable organizations in Dublin cannot be overstated. Prunty, *Dublin Slums, 1800–1925*, pp.238, 273.

12. A. Davin, 'Imperialism and Motherhood', *History Workshop*, 5 (Spring 1978), pp.9–65; J. Bourke, *Husbandry to Housewifery: Women, Economic Change, and Housework*

in Ireland, 1890–1914 (Oxford: Clarendon Press, 1993). Davin notes that, similarly, in Britain, from the beginning of the twentieth century, child health 'took on a new importance in public discussion, reinforced by emphasis on the value of a healthy and numerous population'. Furthermore, J. Bourke's work has explored how the increasing importance of domestic life in late nineteenth-century Ireland was a precursor of social and national improvement.

13. R. Porter, *The Greatest Benefit to Mankind: A Medical History of Humanity from Antiquity to the Present* (London: Harper Collins, 1997), p.555 and R. Bivins, '"The English Disease" or "Asian Rickets"? Medical Responses to Postcolonial Immigration', *Bulletin of the History of Medicine*, 81, 3 (2007), pp.533–68.

14. Porter, *The Greatest Benefit to Mankind*, p.401. For further information on rickets in nineteenth-century Dublin, see Conor Ward's chapter in this volume.

15. A. Hardy, 'Rickets and the Rest: Child-Care, Diet, and the Infectious Children's Diseases, 1850–1914', *Social History of Medicine*, 5, 3 (1992), pp.389–412.

16. 'Children's Sunshine Home', *Irish Times*, 2 July 1925.

17. G. Jones, *'Captain of all These Men of Death': The History of Tuberculosis in Nineteenth- and Twentieth-Century Ireland* (Amsterdam: Rodopi, 2001), p.79.

18. Prunty, *Dublin Slums, 1800–1925*, p.234.

19. M.E. Daly, *Dublin the Deposed Capital: A Social and Economic History, 1860–1914* (Cork: Cork University Press, 1984), p.266.

20. M.J. Maguire, *Precarious Childhood in Post-Independence Ireland* (Manchester: Manchester University Press, 2001), p.27.

21. Daly, *Dublin, the Deposed Capital*, p.268.

22. Anonymous, *Dublin Explorations and Reflections* (Dublin: Maunsel, 1917), p.29, cited in K.C. Kearns, *Dublin Tenement Life: An Oral History* (Dublin: Gill & Macmillan, 2006), p.36.

23. Kearns, *Dublin Tenement Life*, p.36.

24. Ibid., p.140.

25. C. Steedman, 'Bodies, Figures and Physiology: Margaret McMillan and the Late Nineteenth-Century Remaking of Working-Class Childhood', in R. Cooter (ed.), *In the Name of the Child: Health and Welfare, 1880–1940* (Basingstoke: Routledge, 1992), p.35.

26. 'Crippled Children', *British Medical Journal (BMJ)*, 2, 3436 (1926), p.905.

27. D. Price, 'Memorandum on the Sunshine Home, Stillorgan', dated 1 July 1953 (Overend Archive, Airfield Trust, Dublin); see also Anne Mac Lellan's chapter in this volume.

28. Letter of appeal, May 1925 (Overend Archive, Airfield Trust, Dublin).

29. 'Obituary: Dr Ella Webb', *Irish Times*, 26 August 1946.

30. 'Obituary: Dr Ella Webb', *BMJ*, 2, 4470 (1946), p.348.

31. *St Stephen's*, 2, 8 (December 1905), p.182.

32. 'Obituary: Dr Ella Webb', *Irish Times*, 26 August 1946.

33. 'Obituary: Dr Ella Webb', p.348.

34. N. Kearney and C. Skehill (eds), *Social Work in Ireland: Historical Perspectives* (Dublin: Institute of Public Administration, 2005), p.166.

35. 'Obituary: Dr Ella Webb', p.348.

36. E. Ovenden, 'Medicine', in M. Bradshaw (ed.), *Open Doors for Irishwomen: A Guide to the Professions Open to Educated Women in Ireland* (Dublin: Irish Central Bureau for the Employment of Women, 1907), p.36.

37. O. Walsh, *Anglican Women in Dublin: Philanthropy, Politics and Education in the Early Twentieth Century* (Dublin: UCD Press, 2005), p.95.

38. See M. Luddy, *Women and Philanthropy in Nineteenth-Century Ireland* (Cambridge: Cambridge University Press, 1995).

39. Walsh, *Anglican Women in Dublin*, p.4.

40. M. Ó hÓgartaigh, *Kathleen Lynn: Irishwoman, Patriot, Doctor* (Dublin: Irish Academic Press, 2006), p.68.

41. Kelly, *Irish Women in Medicine*, p.163.

42. 'Medical Inspection of School Children', *BMJ*, 1, 2785 (1914), p.1094.

43. Kelly, *Irish Women in Medicine, c. 1880s–1920s*, p.165.

44. Ibid., p.52.

45. Jones, *'Captain of all These Men of Death'*, p.101.

46. The Countess of Aberdeen (ed.), *Ireland's Crusade against Tuberculosis: Vol. 1: The Plan of Campaign: Being a Series of Lectures Delivered at the Tuberculosis Exhibition, 1907, under the Auspices of the Women's National Health Association of Ireland* (Dublin: Maunsell, 1908), p.5.

47. Davin, 'Imperialism and Motherhood', p.12.

48. Ó hÓgartaigh, *Kathleen Lynn*, pp.75–6.

49. 'Tuberculosis Exhibition in Bray', *Irish Times*, 27 March 1909. For more on Lady Aberdeen's work in Ireland, see A. Evans, 'The Countess of Aberdeen's Health Promotion Caravans', *Journal of the Irish Colleges of Physicians and Surgeons*, 24, 3 (July 1995), pp.211–18.

50. Aberdeen, *Ireland's Crusade against Tuberculosis*, p.7.

51. Advertisement for Jessel's cod liver oil extract tablets, *Nenagh Guardian*, 5 February 1944.

52. Advertisement for Scott's emulsion, *Weekly Irish Times*, 25 February 1911.

53. R.D. Apple, *Vitamania: Vitamins in American Culture* (New Brunswick, NJ: Rutgers University Press, 1996), p.27.

54. 'War on the Slums', letter to the editor, *Irish Times*, 20 July 1931.

55. E. Webb, 'Ten Years' Work at the Children's Sunshine Home, Stillorgan', *Irish Journal of Medical Science (IJMS)*, 10, 5 (1935), pp.225–9.

56. Ibid.

57. E. Watson, *The Children's Sunshine Home: A Success Story* (Dublin: Brunswick Press, 1988), p.5.

58. 'The Cure of Rickets: Home to be Established near Dublin', *Freeman's Journal*, 24 June 1923, p.8.

59. Watson, *The Children's Sunshine Home*, p.5.

60. 'Children's Sunshine Home', *Irish Times*, 2 July 1925.

61. 'Children's Sunshine Home, Stillorgan', *Irish Times*, 13 August 1925.

62. Ibid.

63. 'The Children's Hope', *Dublin Evening Mail*, 5 June 1924, from Scrapbook of Newspaper Cuttings (Overend Archive, Airfield Trust, Dublin).

64. Jones, '*Captain of all These Men of Death*', p.140.

65. Ibid.

66. Ibid., p.141.

67. E.G. Webb and L.A. Baker, 'First Annual Report of the Dublin Pasteurised Milk Depot', *Dublin Journal of Medical Science*, 129, 1 (1910), pp.59–65.

68. 'Subscriptions and Appeals: The Children's Sunshine Home', *Irish Times*, 2 August 1924.

69. For example, in 1942 the home received £722 from donations, bequests and collections, while in 1943 it received £1,197 (Annual Reports of the Children's Sunshine Home, 1942 and 1943, Overend Archive, Airfield Trust, Dublin).

70. Appeal leaflet, 1927 from Scrapbook of Newspaper Cuttings (Overend Archive, Airfield Trust, Dublin).

71. Appeal leaflet, 1925 from Scrapbook of Newspaper Cuttings (Overend Archive, Airfield Trust, Dublin).

72. Christmas appeal envelope, 1924 from Scrapbook of Newspaper Cuttings (Overend Archive, Airfield Trust, Dublin).

73. Extract from the Scheme of the Children's Sunshine Home (Overend Archive, Airfield Trust, Dublin).

74. Extract from the Scheme of the Children's Sunshine Home (Overend Archive, Airfield Trust, Dublin).

75. Letter of appeal, May 1925 (Overend Archive, Airfield Trust, Dublin).

76. L. Earner-Byrne, *Mother and Child: Maternity and Child Welfare in Dublin, 1922–60* (Manchester: Manchester University Press, 2007), pp.75–82.

77. Ó hÓgartaigh, *Kathleen Lynn*, p.92.

78. Ibid., pp.92–105.

79.   Earner-Byrne, *Mother and Child*, p.76.

80.   Report of the Children's Sunshine Home for period 1 March 1944 to 28 February 1948 (Overend Archive, Airfield Trust, Dublin).

81.   Webb, 'Ten Years' Work at the Children's Sunshine Home, Stillorgan', pp.225–9.

82.   Ibid.

83.   Jessop, 'Results of Rickets Surveys in Dublin' p.291.

84.   Letter from Mrs D. to Letitia Overend, dated 13 June 1927 (Overend Archive, Airfield Trust, Dublin).

85.   Annual Report of the Children's Sunshine Home for Year 1937–8 (Overend Archive, Airfield Trust, Dublin).

86.   See E.G.A. Webb, 'Calcium Metabolism in Relation to Disease', *IJMS*, 11, 5 (1936), pp.209–19.

87.   'Some Problems of Public Health', *BMJ*, 2, 3908 (1935), p.1069.

88.   D. Price, 'Memorandum on the Sunshine Home, Stillorgan', dated 1 July 1953 (Overend Archive, Airfield Trust, Dublin).

89.   Children's Sunshine Home, Stillorgan, Resolution of 3 December 1930 (Overend Archive, Airfield Trust, Dublin).

90.   Jones, '*Captain of all These Men of Death*', p.142.

91.   Ibid.

92.   G. Jones, *Social Hygiene in Twentieth-Century Britain* (London: Croom Helm, 1986), pp.72–7, cited in L. Bryder, '"Wonderlands of Buttercup, Clover and Daisies": Tuberculosis and the Open-Air School Movement in Britain, 1907–39', in R. Cooter (ed.), *In the Name of the Child: Health and Welfare, 1880–1940* (Basingstoke: Routledge, 1992), p.86.

93.   Letter of appeal, May 1925 (Overend Archive, Airfield Trust, Dublin); Bryder, '"Wonderlands of Buttercup, Clover and Daisies"', p.90.

94.   E. Webb's writings (Overend Archive, Airfield Trust, Dublin).

95.   'Sunshine Home's Work', *Irish Press*, 28 May 1934.

96.   'Good Work at Stillorgan Home', *Irish Independent*, 4 June 1928.

97.   Ibid.

98.   Letter of appeal, May 1925 (Overend Archive, Airfield Trust, Dublin).

99.   'Extension of Sunshine Home', *BMJ*, 1, 3676 (1931), p.1089.

100. Annual Report of the Children's Sunshine Home for Year 1939–40 (Overend Archive, Airfield Trust, Dublin).

101. 'Making Sick Children into Useful Citizens', *Irish Press*, 3 June 1940.

102. Watson, *The Children's Sunshine Home: A Success Story*, p.14.

103. Prunty, *Dublin Slums, 1800–1925*, p.272.

104. 'Making Sick Children into Useful Citizens', *Irish Press*, 3 June 1940.

Chapter 9

1. I. Milne, 'The 1918–19 Influenza Pandemic in Ireland: A Leinster Perspective', (unpublished PhD thesis, Trinity College Dublin, 2011); Eadem, 'Mutant Flu Viruses have killed over 100m', *Irish Independent*, 17 October 2005. The 800,000 estimate of influenza cases is based on the author's own calculations, using a widely accepted death rate of 2.5 per cent of those infected (see for example J.K. Taubenberger, 'The Origin and Virulence of the 1918 "Spanish" Influenza Virus', *Proceedings of the American Philosophical Society*, 150, 1 (March 2006), pp.86–112); the author is grateful to medical statistician Anthony Kinsella who later corroborated this estimate with rather more sophisticated calculations.

2. Researchers from several disciplines have offered reasons why young adults would be particularly prone to becoming ill and dying from this disease. There has been some consensus that deaths in this age group may have been caused by a cytokine storm, an over-reaction of the immune system to an infection, more frequently seen in young, healthy adults with a strong immune system, which has in recent years been observed in young adult H5N1 victims. Perhaps young adults, as the family income earners, would have been more likely to catch the disease by mixing with people at and on their way to work, and may have been forced by economic necessity or family circumstance to return to work before fully recovered, placing themselves at a higher risk of dying from pneumonia. Young adults would also have included parents of young children, so the children may have caught it through close contact with the parents. See Milne, 'The 1918–19 Influenza Pandemic in Ireland: A Leinster Perspective'.

3. In the first published work on the pandemic's effects in Ireland, Caitriona Foley wrote that 'children were spared while their parents died' and supported this claim by citing a Local Government Board source as saying that infants and the aged were least affected by the disease; she plotted the numbers of influenza deaths by age group on a graph to indicate that the vast majority of deaths occurred in the 25–35 age group. C. Foley, *The Last Irish Plague* (Dublin: Irish Academic Press, 2011), pp.29–34. My statistical analysis shows that in fact children under 5 were almost as vulnerable to dying from the disease as adults in the 25–35 age group, when the deaths are plotted per thousand of the estimated living population, and that children under 5 were statistically far more likely to die from this disease than older children, when the deaths in these age categories were plotted in the same way.

4. *Fifty-Fifth Annual Report of Registrar-General for Ireland for 1918 (Births, Deaths, and Marriages)* (1919), x, cmd. 450. *Fifty-Sixth Annual Report of Registrar-General for Ireland for 1919 (Births, Deaths, and Marriages)* (1920), xi, cmd. 997. Some factors that suggest that influenza deaths were not all certified: reports of mass influenza graves in Leixlip and Naas; lack of death certification for people understood to have died from influenza;

newspaper reports that do not tally with weekly death reports from the registrar general; the Local Government Board admitted in its annual report that influenza statistics were under-recorded in the report, *Forty-Seventh Annual Report of the Local Government Board for Ireland for the Year ended 31 March 1919* (1920), xxi, cmd. 578.

5. R. Aronowitz, 'Lyme Disease: The Social Construction of a New Disease and its Social Consequences', *Milbank Quarterly*, lxix, 1 (1991), pp.79–112.

6. Between 1916 and 1923, Ireland was in a transitional status, moving from political union with Britain towards a limited independence as a British dominion. There were three distinct phases to the revolutionary period, beginning with the 1916 rebellion, followed by the War of Independence (1919–21) and the Civil War (1922–3); see D. Ferriter, *The Transformation of Ireland, 1900-2000* (London: Profile Books, 2004) *passim*. Some of the key political events of the period coincided with the influenza period. The connection between the influenza and the political situation is well known, having been written about in contemporary newspapers, in political memoirs by F. Gallagher in *The Four Glorious Years, 1918-1921* (Dublin: Blackwater Press, 2005; 1st edn 1953, under *nom de plume* D. Hogan), R. Brennan in *Allegiance* (Dublin: Browne & Nolan, 1950) and *Doctor* (Dublin: Irish Academic Press, 2006), and more recently in M. Ó hÓgartaigh, *Kathleen Lynn: Irishwoman, Patriot, Doctor* (Dublin: Irish Academic Press, 2006), G. Beiner, P. Marsh and I. Milne, 'Greatest Killer of the Twentieth Century: The Great Flu in 1918–19', *History Ireland* (March/April 2009), pp.40–3, H. Ó Brolcháin, *All in the Blood* (Dublin: A. & A. Farmar, 2006), C. Foley, *Last Irish Plague*, W. Murphy, 'The Tower of Hunger: Political Imprisonment and the Irish, 1910–1921' (unpublished PhD thesis, University College Dublin, 2006), P. Marsh, 'The Effects of the 1918–19 Influenza Pandemic on Ulster' (unpublished PhD thesis, Queen's University Belfast, 2010) and Milne, 'The 1918–19 Influenza Pandemic in Ireland: A Leinster perspective'.

7. These interviews, conducted as part of the author's doctoral research, remain stored in her personal archive.

8. J. Bornat, 'Oral History as a Social Movement: Reminiscence and Older People', in R. Perks and A. Thomson (eds), *The Oral History Reader* (London: Routledge, 1998), pp.189–205.

9. C. Rosenberg, *Explaining Epidemics and Other Studies in the History of Medicine* (Cambridge: Cambridge University Press, 1992), p.283.

10. Interview with R.B. McDowell, Trinity College Dublin, in January 2007.

11. Many authorities cite good nursing as being the most effective treatment for this influenza. See for example P. Marsh, 'Aid for the Poor in Ulster during the Influenza Pandemic of 1918–19', in P. Gray and V. Crossman (eds), *Poverty and Welfare in Ireland, 1838-1948* (Dublin: Irish Academic Press, 2011).

12. Milne, 'The 1918–19 Influenza Pandemic in Ireland: A Leinster Perspective'.

13. Interview with Elizabeth Molloy, Lucan, County Dublin, February 2007.

14. R.B. McDowell, *Crisis and Decline: The Fate of the Southern Unionists* (Dublin: Lilliput Press, 1997); R.B. McDowell, *McDowell on McDowell: A Memoir* (Dublin: Lilliput Press, 2008). McDowell was interviewed for *Outbreak*, a documentary series on epidemic disease produced by Janet Gallagher, RTÉ 1, 2 June 2009.

15. Interview with Catherine Doyle, Lucan, County Dublin, February 2007.

16. Miss Doyle (her preferred mode of address) referred to bodies turning black. The occurrence of heliotrope cyanosis was regarded by doctors as a sign of imminent death. It happened as the tiny air sacs in the lungs, the alveoli, filled with blood and other body fluids, causing them to harden into a consolidated mass; as the alveoli filled, the amount of oxygen pumped into the blood was reduced, turning it from a healthy oxygenated red to a distinctly unhealthy shade of purple, which gave the skin a mauve colour; when life ended, the body turned black. M. Honigsbaum, *Living with Enza* (Basingstoke: Macmillan, 2009), pp.24–5.

17. Personal communication with Kathleen McMenamin, née O'Connor, Rathmullan, County Donegal, October 2010.

18. Interview with Olive Vaughan, née Burgess, in Brabazon Nursing Home, St John's Road, Sandymount, Dublin, January 2007.

19. Interview with Enid, name and address with author, July 2007.

20. Interview with Tommy Christian, Ardclough, County Kildare, April 2007. *Outbreak*, produced by Janet Gallagher, RTÉ 1, 2 June 2009.

21. Lord Cloncurry's diary for 1918 and 1919. In local hands. Entry for Monday 28 October 1918: 'At Lyons, dry day all hands at lifting and pitting potatoes in Skeagh. Nine of the workmen away from work, mainly influenza. Ten women and girls from Celbridge picking potatoes.'

22. Interview with Tommy Christian, November 2007.

23. Some medical doctors placed emphasis on purging the bowels as part of the influenza treatment regime. Tommy's reference to gruel probably alludes to this.

24. Interview with Nellie's son, Jim Tubridy, Cooraclare, County Clare, November 2008.

25. Interview with Lena Higgins in Larchfield Nursing Home, Naas, County Kildare, July 2007.

26. Interview with Sister Theresa Connaghton, Sancta Maria Dominican Nursing Home, Cabra Road, Dublin, March 2007.

27. Interview with Sister Wilfrid Callanan. Sancta Maria Dominican Nursing Home, Cabra Road, Dublin, March 2007.

28. R.B. McDowell died on 28 August 2011, aged 97. An obituary in the *Daily Telegraph* noted his 'terror of draughts' (31 August 2011); he was frequently to be seen walking

around Trinity College in an overcoat and a long woolly scarf, even in summer, perhaps a legacy of his early illness.

29. See for example J. Colgan and D. Cormack, 'Leixlip–Confey Gravestones', *Journal of the County Kildare Archaeological Society*, 19, 3 (2004–5), p.502.

Chapter 10

1. The seminal text with regard to tuberculosis in Ireland remains G. Jones, '*Captain of all These Men of Death': The History of Tuberculosis in Nineteenth- and Twentieth-Century Ireland* (Amsterdam: Rodopi, 2001). Recent published works on tuberculosis include F. Condrau and M. Worboys (eds), *Tuberculosis Then and Now: Perspectives on the History of an Infectious Disease* (Montreal, Kingston, London and Ithaca: McGill-Queen's University Press, 2010); S. Kirby, 'Sputum and the Scent of Wallflowers: Nursing in Tuberculosis Sanatoria 1920–1970', *Social History of Medicine*, 23, 3 (December 2010), pp.602– 20; S. Kelly, '"Suffer the Little Children": Childhood Tuberculosis in the North of Ireland, c. 1865 to 1965' (unpublished PhD thesis, University of Ulster, 2008); A. Mac Lellan, '"That Preventable and Curable Disease": Dr Dorothy Price and the Eradication of Tuberculosis in Ireland, 1930–60' (unpublished PhD thesis, University College Dublin, 2011).

2. Much of the recent writing on children with regard to tuberculosis concentrates on pre-tubercular children, such as C. Connolly, *Saving Sickly Children: The Tuberculosis Preventorium in American Life, 1909–1970* (New Brunswick, NJ: Rutgers University Press, 2008); T. Rymin, '"Tuberculous-Threatened Children": The Rise and Fall of a Medical Concept in Norway, c. 1900–1960', *Medical History*, 52, 3 (July 2008), pp.347–64. Recent works that consider children with active tuberculosis are: A. Shaw and C. Reeves, *The Children of Craig-y-nos: Life in a Welsh Sanatorium, 1922–1959* (Milton Keynes: Wellcome Trust Centre for the History of Medicine, 2009) and S. Kelly, 'Education of Tubercular Children in Northern Ireland, 1921 to 1955', *Social History of Medicine*, 24, 2 (August 2011).

3. Jones, '*Captain of all These Men of Death'*, p.230, source Public Record Office of Northern Ireland (PRONI), TBA 6/9/2. Committee of Enquiry (provisional figures):

	NI	Eng. & Wales	Scotland	Éire
1922	166	112	119	153
1940	98	70	82	125
1945	80	62	79	124
1953	23	20	26	40

4. See Jones, 'Captain of all These Men of Death' for full discussion of the factors that influenced the tuberculosis epidemic in Ireland.

5. The author recorded fifty-three oral history interviews with regard to experience of tuberculosis. Ten of the interviewees had personal experience of bone and joint tuberculosis. An eleventh interview was carried out by email. Oral history interviewee 1 (OH1) (year of birth (yob) 1931), OH3A (yob 1942), OH13 (yob 1925), OH26 (yob 1940), OH31 (yob 1922), OH32 (yob 1941), OH38 (yob 1931), OH40 (yob 1947), OH43 (yob 1942), OH53 (yob 1957), personal correspondence with Jonathan Aitken, 17 April 2012 (yob 1942).

6. T.N. Kelynack (ed.), *Tuberculosis in Infancy and Childhood* (London: Balliere, Tindall & Cox, 1908), pp.xi–xiii. Dr Theophilus Nicholas Kelynack (1866–1944) was a physician with particular interest in tuberculosis (Hon. Physician to Mount Vernon Hospital for Consumption and Diseases of the Chest) and child health.

7. OH 26.

8. The history of clean milk can be read in P.J. Atkins, 'White Poison? The Social Consequences of Milk Consumption, 1850-1930', *Social History of Medicine*, 5, 2 (1992), pp.207–27. See also K. Waddington, 'To Stamp Out "So Terrible a Malady": Bovine Tuberculosis and Tuberculin Testing in Britain, 1890–1939', *Medical History*, 48, 1 (2004), pp.29–48. From the 1870s there was growing debate about whether the meat from diseased cattle posed a threat to man. Research in this area was intensified after the International Tuberculosis Congress of 1901 and proved that bacilli of bovine origin could infect the human. This created a consensus that bovine tuberculosis was a public health threat that could and should be tackled. The use of tuberculin as a means to detect tuberculosis in cattle received official support from the Royal Commission on Tuberculosis of 1896 to 1898, and in 1908 Clemens von Pirquet developed a tuberculin test for human use. Whereas previously children were either seen as well or unwell, now they could be shown to have been infected by an organism but not suffering from active disease. They were now defined as 'pre tubercular', and a whole movement attempted to improve their health and prevent them moving into the tubercular category. See note 2 above regarding pre-tubercular children. Kelly, 'Suffer the little Children', pp.87, 93–4.

9. R. Conry, *Flowers of the Fairest* (Dingle: Brandon, 2002), p.19.

10. *Corporation of Belfast Tuberculosis Department Report of the Chief Tuberculosis Officer* (1918), incorporated in the report of the Acting Medical Superintendent of the Municipal Sanatorium, Whiteabbey (1918), pp.28–32. The staff did recommend that they should stay longer.

11. *Corporation of Belfast Tuberculosis Department Report of the Chief Tuberculosis Officer* (1922), p.6.

12. This will be referred to in this chapter as Graymount, and Greenisland when it moved site in 1941 following the Belfast blitz.

13. *Corporation of Belfast Tuberculosis Department Report of the Chief Tuberculosis Officer* (1922), p.19.

14. PRONI, *Belfast Corporation Borough Council, Tuberculosis Committee Minutes*, LA7/9AE/6, 4 June 1923, p.350.

15. A few were chest X-rays but the majority were skeletal. The number of X-rays per child increased faster than the expansion of bed numbers. The hospital had beds for 58 children in 1927; this dropped to 46 beds in 1941 after the move to Greenisland but increased to 120 in 1950.

16. *Northern Ireland Tuberculosis Authority Annual Report* (1952), p.48.

17. *Northern Ireland Tuberculosis Authority Annual Report* (1955), p.52.

18. E. Pearce, *A Textbook of Orthopaedic Nursing* (London: Faber & Faber, 1939), p.131.

19. N.S. Martin, 'Tuberculosis of the Spine: A Study of the Results of Treatment during the last Twenty-Five Years', *Journal of Bone and Joint Surgery*, 52, 4 (November 1970), pp.614–15.

20. For example, OH13, OH32, OH38, OH26.

21. Eight patients – Hip TB: OH 26, OH38, OH43, OH3A; TB spine: OH32, OH40, OH53, OH13. Excluded OH31, who had TB hip and spine.

22. PRONI, Graymount/Greenisland School Roll Book (SCH/535/2/1-5, SCH/534/2/1-24) and OH38.

23. OH26.

24. These will be referred to as Cappagh Hospital and Graymount Hospital.

25. *Belfast Telegraph*, 12 July 1922.

26. Ibid.

27. Ibid.

28. RTÉ Radio 1, Documentary on One: 'Children on the Veranda', 15 February 2009. Interview with R. Conry.

29. OH43.

30. RTÉ Radio 1, 'Children on the Veranda'.

31. Shaw and Reeves, *The Children of Craig-y-nos*, p.53, Interview with Christine Thornton.

32. Pearce, *Textbook of Orthopaedic Nursing*, p.122.

33. Conry, *Flowers of the Fairest*, p.21.

34. OH43.

35. OH32.

36. Ibid.

37. Ibid.
38. RTÉ Radio 1, 'Children on the Veranda'.
39. Conry, *Flowers of the Fairest*, p.30.
40. RTÉ Radio 1, 'Children on the Veranda'.
41. Conry, *Flowers of the Fairest*, p.30.
42. Personal communication with the author from J. Aitken, 17 April 2012.
43. OH38.
44. Pearce, *Textbook of Orthopaedic Nursing*, p.187.
45. J.S. Loughridge, 'Tuberculosis of Joints', *Ulster Medical Journal*, 2, 2 (April 1933), p.111.
46. H.P. Malcolm, 'Hip-Joint Disease', *Ulster Medical Journal*, 2, 4 (October 1933), p.299.
47. A. Borsay, *Disability and Social Policy in Britain since 1750* (Basingstoke: Palgrave Macmillan, 2005), p.55. Quoting from Princess Elizabeth Orthopaedic Hospital, Exeter, Hospital Management and Other Committee Minutes, 16 May 1929.
48. Martin, *Journal of Bone and Joint Surgery*, p.628.
49. OH26.
50. Jones, *'Captain of all These Men of Death'*, p.227.
51. Martin, *Journal of Bone and Joint Surgery*, p.620.
52. Private uncatalogued archive material at Musgrave Park Hospital, previously unviewed.
53. See Musgrave Park Hospital archive.
54. Ibid.
55. H.J. Sneddon, 'Treatment of Tuberculous Disease of the Spine', *Proceedings of the Royal Society of Medicine*, 31, 8 (1938), p.951.
56. PRONI, Belfast Corporation County Borough Council, Minutes of Tuberculosis Committee, LA7/9AE/8, 18 March 1931, p.398.
57. See Musgrave Park Hospital archive.
58. Martin, *Journal of Bone and Joint Surgery*, p.628.
59. Calculated by author from Registrar General (Ireland) figures.
60. Northern Ireland Tuberculosis Authority annual reports (1947 to 1958).
61. Registrar General (Ireland) mortality figures.
62. OH32.
63. J. Aitken, *Pride and Perjury* (London and New York: Continuum, 2000), p.95.
64. OH38.
65. As mentioned in the interviews of OH 53, OH40, OH38, OH26, OH32.
66. J. Bowlby, *Maternal Care and Mental Health* (Geneva: World Health Organization, 1951); J. Robertson, *Young Children in Hospital* (London: Tavistock Publications, 1958).
67. Conry, *Flowers of the Fairest*, p.8.
68. RTÉ Radio One, 'Children on the Veranda'.

69. J. Aitken, *The American Spectator*, December 2009/January 2010, p.77.

70. RTÉ Radio One, 'Children on the Veranda'.

71. A. Shaw, Craig-y-nos blogspot, http://craig-y-nos.blogspot.co.uk/2009/09/jonathain-aitken-and-tb.html, accessed 1 February 2012.

72. S.K. Kelly, 'Stigma and Silence: Oral Histories of Tuberculosis', *Oral History*, 39, 1 (Spring 2011), pp.65–76.

73. After the introduction of chemotherapy there were forty-three patients from the Musgrave Park coterie who were discharged in as little as six months.

74. Health Protection Agency figures for 2006 show Northern Ireland having the lowest rate of tuberculosis in the United Kingdom.

75. All were from the British Asian community.

76. T. Holland, M. Sangster, R. Paton and L. Omerod, 'Bone and Joint Tuberculosis in Children in the Blackburn Area since 2006: A Case Series', *Journal of Children's Orthopaedics*, 4, 1 (February 2010), pp.67–71.

Index